Exacerbation of Asthma in Children and Exposure to Environmental Tobacco Smoke – A Detailed Review of the Epidemiological Evidence

EXACERBATION OF ASTHMA IN CHILDREN AND EXPOSURE TO ENVIRONMENTAL TOBACCO SMOKE – A DETAILED REVIEW OF THE EPIDEMIOLOGICAL EVIDENCE

PETER N. LEE
AND
BARBARA A. FOREY

Nova Science Publishers, Inc.
New York

For permission to use material from this book please contact us:
Telephone 631-231-7269; Fax 631-231-8175
Web Site: http://www.novapublishers.com

Library of Congress Cataloging-in-Publication Data
ISBN: 978-1-60692-083-1

Published by Nova Science Publishers, Inc. ✢ New York

CONTENTS

List of Tables

Abbreviations

AQOL	Asthma-related (or asthma specific) quality of life
BHR	Bronchial hyperreactivity
BTS	British Thoracic Society
CCR	Cotinine/creatinine ratio
CI	Confidence interval
COHb	Carboxyhaemoglobin
EPA	Environmental Protection Agency
ER	Emergency room or department
ETS	Environmental tobacco smoke
$FEF_{x\%}$	Forced expiratory flow at x% of forced vital capacity
FEV_1	Forced expiratory volume in 1 second
FVC	Forced vital capacity
GP	General practitioner
HDM	House dust mite
ICS	Inhaled corticosteroids
IgE	Immunoglobulin E
IRR	Incidence rate ratio
MMEFR	Mid-maximal expiratory flow rate
NHANES III	Third National Health and Nutrition Examination Survey
NIH	National Institutes of Health (USA)
NK	Not known
NOS	Not otherwise specified
NS	Not significant
OR	Odds ratio

PC_{20} (or PD_{20})	Provocative concentration (or dose) of histamine or methacholine to produce a 20% increase in FEV_1
PEFR	Peak expiratory flow rate
PNLSC	P.N. Lee Statistics and Computing Ltd.
RR	Relative risk
SD	Standard deviation
SE	Standard error
SES	Socio-economic status
SPT	Skin prick test
SRAW	Specific airway resistance
URI	Upper respiratory tract infection

PREFACE

The objective of the work described in this book is to review the epidemiological evidence in children relating ETS exposure to exacerbation of asthma. For a wider review of ETS exposure and asthma, including evidence on exacerbation of asthma from chamber studies, as well as epidemiological evidence on exacerbation of asthma in adults and on asthma induction in children and adults, see Lee and Forey (2007).

Asthma is characterized by episodic symptoms and variable airflow obstruction that occur either spontaneously or in response to environmental exposures. Individuals may be asthmatic or non-asthmatic, the asthmatic state implying the propensity for an asthmatic attack. An agent may "induce" the asthmatic state, causing an individual previously classified as non-asthmatic to be reclassified as asthmatic. An agent may also "exacerbate" asthma, by causing an attack in a known asthmatic or by increasing the severity of symptoms of asthma.

Environmental tobacco smoke (ETS) exposure, or passive smoking, is the inhalation of tobacco smoke other than by puffing on a cigarette, cigar or pipe. ETS consists in the main part of sidestream smoke, emitted from the burning cigarette between puffs, and exhaled mainstream smoke, emitted from the smoker following each puff. Smoking by the mother in pregnancy (*in utero* exposure to maternal smoking) is not ETS exposure as such, as it does not involve inhalation of smoke by the fetus.

Our review considers epidemiological studies that relate indices of ETS exposure to endpoints that concern asthma severity or exacerbation in asthmatic children. No restriction has been made on smoking status, though many of the studies were based on children so young that smoking would effectively be ruled out, and some studies restricted attention to children who had never smoked, smoked no more than a minimum amount or did not currently smoke. Endpoints considered include hospitalization, emergency room (ER) visits and urgent consultations, restricted activity, acute and non-acute asthma, asthma medication, health contacts for asthma, asthma severity, asthma symptoms and acute epidodes, and quality of life and general health, as well as lung function and bronchial responsiveness.

Chapter 1, "The Studies", starts by summarizing the number of relevant publications and studies found, giving reasons why certain publications that seemed possibly relevant were not in fact considered. Then, for each study in turn, there follows a description of the study, including its design, location, number of subjects, and age, sex and smoking status of the subjects, and also a summary of the results. Next follows a summary of the main features of the combined set of studies.

Chapter 2, "The Results", summarises the results by endpoint and shows whether an association has been demonstrated convincingly.

Finally, Chapter 3, "Summary and Conclusions", brings all the material together also including a section which considers other published reviews of the evidence.

Chapter 1

1. THE STUDIES

1.1. INTRODUCTION

Attempts were made to collect all relevant literature published up to and including 2004. Relevant literature was obtained from the extensive files on smoking and health accumulated by P.N. Lee Statistics and Computing Ltd. (PNLSC), from Medline searches, from the references of papers obtained, and from the references of other published reviews. Studies published only as abstracts were included. It was considered more important to obtain all the relevant evidence than to restrict attention unnecessarily to papers published in peer reviewed journals. Papers that were found to contain relevant data were classified into separate studies, taking account that some papers described results from more than one study and that results from some studies were described in multiple publications.

The literature searches identified 60 publications which together described the results of a total of 47 relevant epidemiological studies in children. 18 of the studies were conducted in the USA, four in Canada, 13 in Europe (in a total of 10 countries), five in Turkey or the Middle East, three in India or the Far East, three in Africa and one in New Zealand. Seven references were published as abstracts.

A further 17 publications described studies that seemed possibly relevant, but did not meet the inclusion criteria. The reasons for rejection included no actual data collected on ETS exposure, the study only reporting on whether tobacco smoke brought on wheezing (Speer, 1968), no results reported relating ETS exposure to aggravation of asthma (Wood et al., 1993; Huss et al., 1994; Chadwick, 1996; Gilliland et al., 2001; Morgan et al., 2004), results not reported separately for children (Tarlo et al., 2000; Bayona et al., 2002), results not reported separately for asthmatics (Lebowitz, 1984a; Lebowitz, 1984b; Toyoshima et al., 1987; Strachan et al., 1990; Agudo et al., 1994; Henderson et al., 1995; Fielder et al., 1999; Willers et al., 2000) and endpoint (respiratory illness) too broad (Gilliland et al., 2003). A further study (Bener et al., 1991) was rejected as the data presented seemed totally implausible, with 85% of a sample of schoolchildren reported to have asthma and the odds of having a frequent attack 34 times higher if one of the parents smoked.

The studies are described individually in sections 1.2 (USA), 1.3 (Canada), 1.4 (Europe), 1.5 (Asia) and 1.6 (Other). Section 1.7 then summarizes various relevant aspects of the studies considered and section 2 brings together the findings by type of endpoint.

1.2. Description of the Studies – USA

The Minnesota Study

O'Connell and Logan (1974) collected information from 400 asthmatic children aged 2 to 16 years (60% male) on whether smoking induced or aggravated their asthma. For 37 children whose parents' smoking was considered to have a significantly adverse effect on their asthma, it was recommended as a part of treatment that this exposure be eliminated, and 35 were available for follow-up six months to two years later. By then, the asthma had improved in 90% (18/20) of children where parents had stopped smoking and in 27% (4/15) where parents had continued. The relative risk can be estimated as 3.38 (1.44-7.91). Results on whether smoking irritated the respiratory tract were also presented for 228 children without asthma, allergic rhinitis or atopic dermatitis and whose siblings had no allergic disease. This study has some weaknesses. It uses endpoints which are rather soft and poorly defined, and it is hard to tell whether responses relate to tobacco smoke in general or to the parents' smoking. No statistical tests were conducted, though, as shown above, differences by stopping smoking are statistically significant.

The Michigan and Massachusetts Study

In random population surveys of children aged 0-17 conducted in an urban county in Michigan and a rural county in Massachusetts, USA, Gortmaker et al (1982) collected data on the prevalence of asthma and of functionally impairing asthma and on parental smoking, but not on smoking by the child. Although the paper is mainly concerned with prediction of asthma and of function-impairing asthma by various factors including parental smoking, these analyses are not relevant to exacerbation of asthma.

However data were provided which allow one to relate maternal smoking to the probability, among asthmatic children, of the asthma being functionally impairing. This analysis, summarized below, shows a non-significant tendency for the probability to be higher if the mother smokes.

Sample	Functional impairment	Mother non-smoker	Mother smoker	OR (95% CI)
Michigan	No	71	69	
	Yes	20	28	1.44 (0.74-2.79)
Massachusetts	No	11	11	
	Yes	3	4	1.33 (0.24-7.40)
Total (adjusted for sample)	No	82	80	
	Yes	23	32	1.43 (0.79-2.65)

The First New York Study

Evans et al. (1987) studied 276 asthmatic children from low income families, collecting data on smoking by the parents (and by the children themselves), on pulmonary function (at a random clinic visit up to 1 year after interview), on emergency health care use in the year prior to the interview and on various other potential confounding variables. The children were of average age 9.9 years, with 60% male. After eliminating 77 with some data missing and 8 who reported being smokers, the analyses carried out involved 191 children. Compared to children with no smokers in the household, there was no evidence of a significant reduction in pulmonary function in children in households where one or more parents smoked. Indeed mean pulmonary function scores were somewhat higher where a smoker was present (FEV_1 1.60ℓ vs 1.49ℓ; PEFR 3.19ℓ/sec vs 2.74ℓ/sec; $FEF_{25\text{-}75\%}$ 1.60ℓ/sec vs 1.42ℓ/sec). There was also no significant association of household smoking with the mean number of hospitalisations in the year prior to enrolment. Household smoking was, however, significantly associated with an increase in the mean frequency of visits to the emergency room over the last year. The difference was significant whether or not adjustment for the mean number of days with asthma symptoms per month was made (3.46 vs 2.12, $p=0.008$) or was not made (3.09 vs 1.83, $p<0.05$). Frequency of asthma symptoms was not itself associated with household smoking. The strength of the association of household smoking with emergency room visits was unaffected by counting only households with 2 or more smokers as exposed. It is unclear how parental smoking might markedly increase the frequency of emergency room visits without apparently worsening lung function, or increasing symptom prevalence or the frequency of hospitalisation.

The Boston Study

O'Connor et al. (1987) studied the relationship between parental smoking and airway reactivity in 286 children, including 21 asthmatics (mean age 12 years, 62% male) none of whom smoked themselves. Nine had a mother who smoked. Compared to the other 12 asthmatics, those with a smoking mother had a lower mean FEV_1 (100.8% vs 102.9%) and $FEF_{25\text{-}75\%}$ (76.1% vs 85.8%) and a higher mean FVC (107.8% vs 104.0%) as a percentage of predicted, none of these differences being statistically significant. Following cold air challenge, the response (fall in FEV_1 following challenge expressed as a percentage of predicted FEV_1) was almost significantly higher when the mother smoked (24.0 vs 11.9, p=0.07). Using linear regression to adjust for predicted FEV_1 this difference became significant (p=0.02). Adjustment for other independent variables in a multiple regression analysis did not affect this conclusion. Paternal smoking was unrelated to bronchial responsiveness to cold air. The small sample size and the marginal nature of the significance reported limit interpretation of these findings.

The Second New York Study

In an abstract Lilienfeld et al. (1990) briefly described results of a study of inner city children aged 3-14 years, comparing 72 acute asthmatics in a hospital emergency room and 35 non-acute asthmatics attending an asthma clinic. Urinary cotinine/creatinine ratio (CCR) was used as an index of ETS exposure, the acute asthmatics having a non-significantly lower frequency of a ratio greater than 30 ng/mg (OR 0.92, p=0.85). Household smoking was also determined by questionnaire but results comparing these two groups were not given in the abstract. The authors concluded that *"recent smoke exposure is not the trigger of the acute attack."*

The results were later described more fully (Ehrlich et al., 1992). The groups of acute and non-acute asthmatics were reported to be of similar age (range 3-14 years), sex (62% male) and socio-economic status (SES), all the children being non-smokers. African-American children were somewhat over-represented in the acute group (37% vs 26%), but not significantly. The acute asthmatics were significantly more likely to have had a recent upper respiratory infection (URI) (OR 2.5, 95% CI 1.1-5.6), and to have previously used the emergency room (97% vs 86%, p=0.02). Interestingly they were less likely to have previously attended an asthma clinic (65% vs 100%, p<0.001), or use daily asthma medication (36% vs 80%, p<0.001). As shown below, the groups did not differ on ETS exposure variables.

The authors noted that *"we were unable to show an effect of passive smoke exposure on the precipitation of acute asthmatic effects."*

	Asthma		
ETS exposure variable	Acute	Non-Acute	OR (95% CI)
Any smoker at home	53%	57%	0.84 (0.37-1.89)
Cigs/day by all smokers	7.7	10.7	Not significant
Maternal caregiver smokes	40%	51%	0.64 (0.28-1.44)
CCR[1] ≥ 30 ng/mg	38%	39%	0.90 (0.39-2.06)
Mean CCR (ng/mg)	46.2	38.5	Not significant
Number of subjects	72	35	

[1] CCR = cotinine/creatinine ratio.

National Health Interview Survey

In an analysis based on 4331 children aged 0-5 years participating in the 1981 US National Health Interview Survey, Weitzman et al. (1990b) presented a table giving, by maternal smoking status in pregnancy, the number of mothers, the prevalence of asthma and the percentage of children using asthma medications. These data can be used to estimate ORs for asthma medication by amount of maternal smoking in pregnancy among asthmatics.

	Maternal smoking in pregnancy (cigs/day)				
	0	1-9	10+	Any	Total
With asthma	74	17	26	43	117
Using asthma medications (%)	16 (21.6)	3 (17.6)	11 (42.3)	14 (32.6)	30 (25.6)
OR (95% CI)	1.00	0.78 (0.20-3.04)	2.66 (1.02-6.91)	1.75 (0.75-4.07)	

These results, which are unadjusted for any potential confounding factor, show some evidence of an association, which is marginally significant ($p<0.05$) for maternal smoking of 10+ cigs/day.

A figure was also presented showing mean number of overnight hospitalisations by maternal smoking in pregnancy, separately for non-asthmatic and asthmatic children. For asthmatic children, the numbers (1.1 for no smoking, 1.3 for 1-9/day and 1.0 for 10+/day) showed no significant relationship.

In a further paper by the same group (Weitzman et al., 1990a) data were presented for children aged 2-5 years on the basis that parents of younger children might mistakenly report respiratory illnesses associated with wheezing as asthma. The following table can be constructed:

	Maternal smoking in pregnancy (cigs/day)	
	None or 1-9	10+
With asthma	76	23
Using asthma medication (%)	14 (18%)	9 (39%)
OR (95% CI)	1.00	2.85 (1.03-7.88)

These data considerably overlap those tabulated previously.

The Portland Study

Chilmonczyk et al. (1993), and previously in an abstract Salmun et al. (1992), reported data for 199 asthmatic children aged up to 13 (72% boys) on smoking by parents and other household members, smoking at day-care, cotinine in urine, number of acute exacerbations of asthma in the past 12 months, lung function (from 145 of the children), serum theophylline (from 63 of the children) and on demographic and other variables. The main finding was a trend towards an increasing number of exacerbations of asthma and decreasing lung function with increasing ETS exposure, whether based on parental reports (no exposure, mother or others smoke, mother and others smoke) or on urinary cotinine adjusted for creatinine (<10, 10-39, >39 ng/mg). The increased risk of asthma exacerbations was significant after adjustment for maternal age and education level, and for the child's age, sex and day-care attendance, with children in the highest exposure group having almost twice the number of exacerbations of the lowest exposure group (change per category of reported exposure 0.83, 95% CI 0.39 to 1.26, and per category of CCR 0.63, 95% CI 0.10 to 1.07). Although the corresponding reductions in FEV_1 were not statistically significant, significant reductions were seen in FEV_1/FVC and $FEF_{25\text{-}75\%}$ for both exposure indices. In children prescribed theophylline, serum theophylline levels were similar in those exposed and unexposed to smoke in the home, suggesting that the two groups followed medical advice similarly.

The authors emphasized the value of urinary cotinine as a marker of ETS exposure, and concluded that their study *"provides further evidence of an association between exposure to environmental tobacco smoke and pulmonary morbidity in children with asthma."* Although data were collected on severity of the underlying disease, no account was made of this in analysis. Did the more ETS exposed children have more attacks because they were exposed more, or because they had more severe disease to start with?

The Baltimore Study

Ogborn et al. (1994) collected urine samples and data on parent-reported ETS exposure from 56 children aged 3-11 (57% male) on two occasions, first when they attended the hospital emergency department during an acute episode of asthma and second 3 to 4 weeks later when free of symptoms of asthma and feeling well. Using matched-pairs analysis no significant difference was seen between the acute and the well visit in urinary cotinine (means 81 vs 77 ng/ml), CCR (93 vs 97 ng/ml) or the proportion with a ratio of 30 ng/ml or above (80% vs 82%). There was also no significant difference in the reported hours of exposure in the past 48 hours (mean 32 vs 32 hours) or the total number of cigarettes smoked at home in the past 24 hours (31 vs 25). There was, however, a significant ($p=0.02$) difference in the amount of exposure:

	Amount of ETS exposure			
	None	A little	Some	A lot
Acutely asthmatic	10	12	16	14
Well	17	13	20	4

The authors believed that *"this difference may have been due to the parent becoming more sensitised to the issue of passive smoke exposure by the study questionnaire itself and perhaps wanting to minimize the reported exposure."* It also seems possible that knowledge of the asthmatic attack may have affected the answers given to this rather subjective question.

The Seattle Study

In a study first reported as an abstract, Abulhosn et al. (1995) followed up 22 children aged 2-9 years who had been hospitalised for asthma. 11 children living in homes where 1 or more parents smoked and 11 living in non-smoking homes were compared. The groups were stated to be *"comparable"* in age, gender and pre-admission National Institutes of Health (NIH) chronic asthma severity score. They were also similar regarding the proportion discharged home on anti-inflammatory and on beta-agonist asthma therapy. Based on data reported by the parents over the four weeks following hospital discharge, the children in smoking homes had more symptomatic days (3.3 vs 1.4, $p<0.05$). The reduction in use of beta-agonist therapy over the period following discharge was also less in these children (from 18.5 to 14.6 vs from 18.5 to 6.3 treatments per week, $p=0.001$). Children in smoking homes also had more symptomatic nights (2.3 vs 1.4) though this was not significant ($p>0.1$). The authors concluded *"that children returning to smoking households following hospitalisation for acute asthma remain more symptomatic despite greater beta-agonist therapy within four weeks after hospital discharge and therefore recover less completely when compared with those children returning to non-smoking homes."*

Two years later, a paper appeared (Abulhosn et al., 1997). Little extra relevant material was presented. It was noted that the 22 children were aged 2-13 (not 2-9 as previously stated), the mean age being 5.2 in both the groups of 11 children being compared. Nine of the children (41%) were boys. The difference in symptomatic days in the 4 week follow-up period arose because eight (73%) of the children in smoking homes had two or more symptomatic days as against 2 (18%) of the children in non-smoking homes. The data on change in use of beta-agonist therapy between weeks 1 and 4 differed from that given earlier, now being from 20.8 to 8.9 doses per week in the group with non-smoking parents and from 15.3 to 18.0 where the parents smoked ($p<0.001$).

The Davis Study

LeSon and Gershwin (1995) studied all asthmatics aged 5-12 years admitted to a medical centre over a 10 year period, excluding patients with cystic fibrosis. Of the 300 children, 55% male, 13 required intubation for their asthma. A wide range of factors possibly related to the odds of intubation were studied. Exposure to secondhand smoking (from parents, family members or room-mates) was reported by 85% of the children who required intubation and by 20% of those who did not, a highly significant (p<0.001) OR of 22.4 (95% CI 7.4-68.0). [From the data presented we estimate a similar OR of 22.2 but a wider confidence interval of 4.8-102.9. However the relationship is still highly significant.] It should be noted that their analysis identified 11 other factors with a significant OR for intubation, 8 with an OR above 6 and highly significant (p<0.001), though none with an OR as high as for secondhand smoke. Despite this, all the analyses were conducted on a one-factor at a time basis, with no attempt to determine which of the factors were independent. As with the Portland study, Chilmonczyk et al. (1993), data were available on severity but not used in analysis.

The Chicago Study

Hu et al. (1997) studied 705 fifth-graders, mainly blacks aged 10 to 11 years. 5% had ever smoked. 167 (51% male) reported having been diagnosed with asthma. Data were presented relating self-reported prevalence of symptoms and medical treatments to maternal smoking habits in pregnancy and in the past week. Among those with physician-diagnosed asthma, maternal smoking could be related to the proportion who took asthma or wheezing medication in the past 2 weeks and the proportion who attended the emergency room for treatment of asthma in the past 12 months (assuming that those who took medication or who attended the emergency room were a subset of those with physician-diagnosed asthma). The proportions taking medication or attending the emergency room were non significantly lower if the mother smoked.

Time of maternal smoking	Type of outcome	Mother did not smoke Outcome		Mother smoked Outcome		OR (95% CI)
		–	+	–	+	
In pregnancy	Took medication in past 2 weeks	25	52	15	21	0.67(0.30-1.52)
In pregnancy	ER in past 12 months	31	46	16	20	0.84(0.38-1.87)
In past week	Took medication in past 2 weeks	18	44	17	28	0.67(0.30-1.52)
In past week	ER in past 12 months	24	38	19	26	0.86(0.40-1.89)

The New Orleans Study

An abstract summarized the results of an intervention trial (El-Dahr et al., 2000) involving 16 households containing 21 smokers (at least one per household and presumably adults) and 18 asthmatic children aged 6-16 with 56% male. In phase 1 of the study the smokers smoked normally for 3 months. In phase 2 smokers received counselling and smoking cessation aids over a 1 month period in order to encourage them to quit and to cease smoking inside the home for 3 months. Although only 2 of the 21 smokers stopped completely, all of them significantly decreased the number of cigarettes smoked in phase II. The number of cigarettes smoked in the home reduced dramatically (from 18.7 to 0.18 cigs/day, $p=0.0001$), as did nicotine levels in the child's bedroom (12.8 to 1.8 $\mu g/m^3$, $p<0.0001$) and in the living rooms (53.1 to 7.3 $\mu g/m^3$, $p<0.0001$), and the cotinine levels of the parents (340.6 to 257.7 ng/ml, $p=0.002$). The cotinine levels of the children (excluding one who was found to be a smoker) did not vary materially (1.7 to 1.5 ng/ml). As regards asthma in the child, there was a significant increase in days with normal sleep (from 85% to 91%, $p<0.01$), days with normal activity (from 90% to 95%, $p<0.05$), days without cough (from 70% to 87%, $p<0.01$) and days without wheeze (from 78% to 85%, $p=0.06$). Total symptom scores decreased from 1.00 to 0.54 ($p<0.05$). Bronchodilator use was stated to have *"decreased in 7/12 (39%),"* data which are mutually inconsistent (7/12=58%) and with no significance test. There is also no statement of significance regarding average daily PEFR, though with increases in 8/15, no change in 6/15 (actually given as 6/35 but presumably a typographical error) and therefore a decrease in 1/15, we estimate p to be <0.05. FEV_1 was noted to have improved significantly ($p<0.0001$) with 15/17 improving, but metacholine results did not vary, with as many improvements as worsenings. The limitation of this study, from a theoretical point of view, is that there was no formal control group. Had households been randomly assigned to receive or not receive cessation advice, one could have excluded the possibility that changes in asthma status may have, for example, been due to changes in the weather.

The First California Study

Based on the first stage (a cross-sectional survey) of a longitudinal study (the Children's Health Study) conducted in southern California, Li et al. (2000) related lung function in 5263 children simultaneously to sex, asthmatic status, maternal smoking in pregnancy ("*in utero* exposure") and household ETS exposure after birth, after adjustment for community, school grade, spirometer, pressure, technician, log (height), age and race. Approximately 68% of the children were fourth-graders aged 7-13 years, 16% were seventh-graders aged 11-15 and 16% were tenth-graders aged 14-19 years. The study included 442 asthmatic boys and 307 asthmatic girls. Only 13 of the 749 asthmatics were smokers themselves.

The main findings of this study were presented in three tables, one studying effects of *in utero* exposure ignoring ETS, one effects of ETS ignoring *in utero* exposure, and the third joint effects. Each table related to four measures of lung function (FVC, FEV_1, FEV_1/FVC and MMEFR) with results given separately for boys and girls and for asthmatic and non-asthmatic children. The results for single effects in asthmatic children are summarized in the table below:

		Percent change in lung function with statistical significance			
Exposure	Sex	FVC	FEV_1	FEV_1/FVC	MMEFR
In utero vs no *in utero*	Boys	-4.3**	-7.1***	-2.9*	-11.3**
	Girls	+3.3*	-0.5	-3.6***	-8.7*
Past ETS vs no ETS	Boys	-2.2	-4.9*	-2.8*	-9.2*
	Girls	+2.5	+2.1	-0.2	+1.4
One current smoker vs no ETS	Boys	-3.3	-3.9	-0.6	-4.0
	Girls	+1.9	+1.1	-0.8	+7.0
Two or more current smokers vs no ETS	Boys	+0.8	-2.9	-3.6	-5.2
	Girls	+5.9*	+2.7	-2.7	-4.2

* $p<0.05$.
** $p<0.01$.
*** $p<0.001$.

It is clear from these results that the evidence of an association was much stronger for *in utero* exposure than for ETS exposure. For *in utero* exposure 7 of the 8 estimates were of an associated reduction in lung function, with 6 of them statistically significant. The significant result for FVC in girls in the reverse direction was the only conflicting finding. For ETS exposure, the results were far less consistent, with no real evidence of any reduction in lung function in girls and significant reductions in boys only seen in relation to past, but not current, ETS exposure.

The joint effect analyses compare lung function in 5 groups:

Group	ETS	*In utero*
1 (reference)	No	No
2	Past	No
3	Current	No
4	No	Yes
5	Any	Yes

Based on these data it is possible to estimate differences associated with ETS where *in utero* exposure is not present (group 1 compared with weighted average of estimates for groups 2 and 3) and where it is present (difference of estimates for groups 4 and 5). These results (again for asthmatic children) are summarized below:

		Percent change in lung function			
Exposure	Sex	FVC	FEV_1	FEV_1/FVC	MMEFR
ETS vs no ETS	Boys	-0.2	-1.4	-1.2	-2.9
(no *in utero* exposure)	Girls	+1.7	+3.0	+1.7	+10.2
ETS vs no ETS	Boys	-2.7	-0.4	+2.2	+3.0
(*in utero* exposure)	Girls	-5.5	-1.1	+4.2	+13.6

While the significance of these individual changes cannot readily be assessed exactly from the data presented, it seems that none of the reductions associated with ETS (adjusted for *in utero* exposure) are statistically significant. Since there are as many increases as reductions in these estimates it seems that the data from this study do not show any evidence of an effect of ETS exposure independent of *in utero* exposure and little consistent evidence of an effect of ETS exposure ignoring *in utero* exposure.

The authors appear to be rather ambivalent about the conclusions of their study. In the abstract they stated *"In summary both in utero exposure to maternal smoking and ETS exposure were associated with persistent deficits in lung function. The effects of in utero exposure were greatest among children with asthma."* However, reading the last paragraph of the discussion, and most of the paper, one gets the impression that *in utero* effects were much more clearly seen and that it was not so clear whether ETS had any effect.

The Second California Study

An intervention trial (Wilson et al., 2001b) involved 87 ETS-exposed children aged 3 to 12 years (51% male) who had been seen for acute asthma in the preceding year. Following collection of baseline information, the children were randomly assigned to receive intervention (n = 44) or usual care (n = 43). The intervention involved three counselling sessions led by a nurse. These included instruction about asthma and its treatment and the role of ETS in exacerbating and sustaining inflammation, and the collection of urine for cotinine estimation, the estimates then being used at the next session as part of a review of progress in eliminating the child's exposure to tobacco smoke. The usual care also involved giving basic information about asthma and its treatment, but with no specific focus on ETS except for a generic statement that it is best avoided for children with asthma. In both groups the adequacy of medication was assessed and the regimen adjusted where necessary. Data collected from both groups at baseline and at 6- and 12-month follow-up visits included demographic characteristics, asthma history and symptoms, medication, ETS exposure, smoking restrictions, cotinine and health care use. Lung function was collected at baseline and 12 months only.

At baseline the groups did not differ significantly ($p<0.05$) in respect of any characteristics measured, although the intervention group was almost significantly more likely to have a maternal caregiver who smoked (61% vs 42%, $p=0.07$). The main results of the study showed for each of various primary and secondary outcomes the results of "unadjusted" and "adjusted" tests of the intervention effect. The "unadjusted" comparisons involved a simple comparison of the values observed at the end of follow-up, while the "adjusted" comparisons took into account differences observed at baseline, so were equivalent to comparing changes in the two groups. The adjusted results, which seem more meaningful, showed a significant ($p=0.03$) reduction in the probability of having more than one acute medical visit in the study year in the intervention compared to control group, the percentage falling from 50.0% in the year before baseline to 29.6% in the study year in the intervention group, but rising from 37.2% to 46.5% in the usual care group. This difference was more significant ($p=0.01$) in those with 12 month cotinine data, i.e. subjects who had stayed in the study.

Although this result sounds impressive, it should be noted that there were no other significant differences. The estimated adjusted intervention effect was in the hoped for direction as regards cotinine level, hospitalisation for asthma in the year, allowance of smoking in the home, activity limitations and nights awakened, but not as regards cigarettes smoked per day at home, symptom-free days or FEV_1

(for example, FEV_1 increased by 3.72% in the intervention group but by more, 5.38%, in the control group).

Although health-care utilization had reduced more in the intervention group than in the control group, this could not be explained by a reduction in ETS exposure (as measured either by cotinine or by reported changes in smoking rules in the home). The authors noted that adjusting for either of the two indicators of ETS exposure did not affect the significant difference in reduction in health care utilization between the two groups. It would have been helpful here to present data showing, for both groups, how change in ETS exposure correlated with change in health-care utilization, but such results were not shown.

While the results seem consistent with the intervention as a whole being effective in reducing the probability of medical visits and perhaps hospitalisations, it is far from demonstrated that the reduction has actually resulted from ETS reduction. It could be, as the authors admitted, that some other part of the intervention nothing to do with ETS had an effect. The study was quite small and it would need a larger study and perhaps one in which attempts were made to *"measure ETS exposure and behavioral and disease outcomes concurrently"* before a clearer picture can be obtained.

NHANES III

In one analysis based on the Third National Health and Nutrition Examination Survey (NHANES III), Mannino et al. (2002) related indicators of asthma severity to serum cotinine level, divided into three groups (0.050 to 0.115 ng/ml = low, 0.116 to 0.639 ng/ml = intermediate, and 0.640 to 20 ng/ml = high, with 0.050 ng/ml the limit of detection and levels >20 ng/ml assumed to indicate tobacco use). 523 children aged 4-16 with physician-diagnosed asthma were involved, 59% male. After adjusting for age, race/ethnicity, SES, family size and parental history of asthma, comparisons were made of children in the high and low cotinine group as regards various indices of asthma severity. As shown below, there was a significant positive association with moderate or severe asthma, a significant *negative* association with any hospitalisation for asthma in the previous year and a non-significant positive association with the other five indices (not all directly associated with asthma). Adjustment had little effect on the estimated ORs, though it did slightly increase and make significant the positive association with moderate or severe asthma, where the unadjusted estimate was 2.5 (0.97-6.2).

Outcome	Proportion (%)[1]	OR (95% CI)[2]
Moderate or severe asthma (symptoms/illness ≥12 days[3])	21.5	2.7 (1.1-6.8)
Severe asthma (symptoms/illness >300 days[3])	14.6	1.9 (0.6-5.7)
Any physician visit for asthma[3]	41.2	1.8 (0.9-3.8)
Any hospitalisation for asthma[3]	5.7	0.2 (0.1-0.5)
FEV_1 < 80% predicted	10.3	5.1 (0.7-40.6)
Less than very good health status	43.6	1.3 (0.7-2.5)
≥6 school absences[3]	44.4	1.8 (0.9-3.6)

[1] Proportion of all children with outcome.
[2] Comparing children with high (0.64-20ng/mL) and low (<0.116ng/mL) cotinine level.
[3] in previous year.

Comparisons were also made of the same two groups in respect of lung function, with adjustment for age, sitting height, sex, race/ethnicity, SES, parental history of allergy or asthma and family size. Three of the four parameters (FEV_1, FVC and MMEF but not FEV_1/FVC ratio) tested showed a significantly lower adjusted level in the children with high cotinine levels.

Comparing children with highest and lowest cotinine levels		
Outcome	Mean effect %	95% CI
FEV_1	-8.1	-14.7 to -3.5
FVC	-5.6	-10.6 to -0.6
FEV_1/FVC	-3.0	-6.5 to +0.5
MMEF	-12.5	-23.0 to -2.0

Results were not presented in detail for children with intermediate cotinine levels. For asthma outcomes the authors noted that ORs (compared to low cotinine) were *"similar"* to those for high cotinine, but were not statistically significant. However children with intermediate cotinine were noted to have *"lung function levels that were similar to the children with low smoke exposure."* Overall the authors concluded that *"Involuntary smoke exposure is associated with increased asthma severity and worsened lung function in a nationally representative group of US children with asthma."* They considered that the negative association of cotinine with hospitalisation in the previous year might have been *"because some parents may have altered their home smoking policies"* in response to the hospitalisation.

Another analysis based on NHANES III (Chapman et al., 2003) involved 309 children aged 8-16 with physician-diagnosed asthma, 60% of whom were male. Children who were current smokers or who had ever smoked 5 or more packs of cigarettes in their lifetime were excluded. Model-predicted lung function values were presented by the number of smokers in the home, separately for each age, for a child of defined age, race/ethnicity, height, body mass, skinfold thickness, use of gas stove, household annual income, pet ownership and physical activity. Expressing these as differences from households with no smokers in the home gives

	Girls		Boys	
	Smokers in home		Smokers in home	
	1	2+	1	2+
FVC (ℓ)	+0.107	-0.075	+0.055	-0.226*
FEV_1 (ℓ)	+0.104	-0.200*	+0.042	-0.219*
$FEF_{25-75\%}$ (ℓ/sec)	+0.065	-0.738**	+0.154	-0.163
FEV_1/FVC (%)	+0.1	-4.2*	-0.1	-1.1
$FEF_{25-75\%}$/FVC (per sec)	-0.022	-0.211**	-0.020	+0.005

* p<0.1.

** p<0.05.

These results show no association of lung function with having one smoker in the home, but some decrease with having two or more smokers in the home, with significantly ($p<0.05$) reduced $FEF_{25-75\%}$ and $FEF_{25-75\%}$/FVC in girls.

The Baltimore and Washington DC Study

The study by Morkjaroenpong et al. (2002) involved 520 children, predominantly African American, of average age 8.2 years, 40% males. The children were all reported to have doctor-diagnosed asthma, recent symptoms or a recent visit to a hospital or emergency department. Analyses compared 153 children with a caregiver who smoked in the home and 367 with no smokers in the household. Children whose primary care giver smoked but not in the home were excluded from the analysis but it is unclear how children where only other household member(s) smoked were treated. At-home ETS exposure was linked to various aspects of asthma morbidity. No significant relationship was found between smoking in the home and nocturnal symptoms, limited physical activity in the past six months, days of work missed by the caregiver in the past 6 months because of the child's asthma or school days missed by the child because of the asthma.

Further analyses were restricted to the 153 children with at-home exposure, dividing them into 71 with "moderate to high" exposure where 10 cigs/day or more were smoked and 82 with low exposure where 1-9 cigs/day were smoked. Again there was no significant association with limited physical activity, days of work missed or school days missed, but there was a significant association with nocturnal symptoms. Compared to the 43 ETS exposed children with mild intermittent symptoms (≤2 nights per month), the 32 with mild persistent symptoms (2-4 nights) [sic] had an OR of 3.4 (95% CI 1.3-8.8) for moderate to high vs low exposure, while the 78 with moderate-severe symptoms (5+ nights) had an OR of 2.3 (1.0-5.1).

These analyses were unadjusted for any potential confounding factor, but in an additional analysis the authors presented results of further analysis of nocturnal symptoms in a model that simultaneously investigated the role of the child's age, caregiver education, asthma primary care and use of anti-inflammatory medications as well as that of moderate to high vs low ETS exposure. Here the authors reported an unadjusted OR for ETS of 2.84 (1.25-6.42) and an adjusted OR of 2.83 (1.22-6.55).

The analysis was stated to relate to *"presence of nocturnal symptoms,"* but *"presence"* was undefined. The previous results seemed to imply that all the children had at least mild intermittent symptoms so it is unclear what the actual definition of the endpoint used was – perhaps it was at least mild persistent symptoms.

The analysis was also unusual in that with three ETS exposure groups – none, low, and high to moderate – it would seem more sensible to compare the second and third groups with the first group, rather than to compare the third with the second. Based on the data in the paper one can calculate the table shown overleaf.

It is interesting that when viewed in this more standard way, the data show no real indication at all of a *positive* association of ETS exposure with nocturnal symptoms or any of the asthma indices considered, the only significant differences seen being the *reduced* nocturnal symptoms and limited physical activity in the low ETS exposure group.

	ETS exposure				
	None	Low		High to moderate	
Nocturnal symptoms (at least mild persistent)					
No	83	30		13	
Yes	283	52		58	
OR (95% CI)	1.00	0.51	(0.30-0.85)	1.31	(0.68-2.50)
Limited physical activity past 6 months					
No	120	38		23	
Yes	243	44		48	
OR (95% CI)	1.00	0.57	(0.35-0.93)	1.03	(0.60-1.77)
Days of work missed in past 6 months because of child's asthma					
Mean	3.5	3.9		2.3	
SD	5.4	15.3		3.0	
p		NS		NS	
School days missed by child because of asthma					
Mean	6.7	6.2		8.4	
SD	9.0	9.9		10.9	
p		NS		NS	

The Denver Study

Wamboldt et al. (2002) obtained data on ETS exposure, asthma and other variables from 152 children with asthma aged 7-18, 57% male, and from their primary parent. Children with a history of more serious medical treatments for asthma (such as 2 or more hospitalisations in last year) were excluded. A number of the asthma variables (such as asthma knowledge and age at onset) were not of interest to this review, but some were. For the 58 children with a smoker in the household (including if the asthmatic child was a smoker), compared to the 94 with no smoker in the household, no significant difference was noted in functional severity or in AQOL as reported by the child. The score for AQOL as reported by the parent was however significantly lower (poorer) (5.38 vs 6.13, $p<0.005$) where there was a smoker in the household. No adjustment was made for any potential confounding variable.

The Third New York Study

A randomized clinical trial conducted in Rochester (Halterman et al., 2004) involved 184 children aged 3 to 7 years (63% male) with mild persistent to severe persistent asthma. They were allocated to either school-based care (daily inhaled corticosteroids [ICS] provided through the school) or a usual-care group (ICS not given through the school). For 180 of the children, data were available on at home ETS exposure and on various outcomes assessed monthly for a year. Based on the combined data from the two groups, the following comparisons can be made by ETS exposure.

Variable	ETS exposure No	ETS exposure Yes	Significance of differences[1]
Number of children	101	79	
No of symptom-free days[2]	10.97	9.69	$p<0.01$
No of symptom days[2]	2.07	3.07	$p<0.01$
No of symptom nights[2]	2.07	3.05	$p<0.01$
No of days using rescue inhaler[2]	1.97	2.51	NS
Overall change in AQOL[3]	0.36	0.55	NS
Total absences from school	5.92	10.28	$p<0.01$
			OR (95% CI)
3+ acute visits	23 (23%)	21 (27%)	1.23 (0.62-2.43)
1+ hospitalisations	6 (6%)	3 (4%)	0.63 (0.15-2.58)

[1] For the first six variables the significance is based on a t-test based on the means and standard deviations provided, although the distribution may not be normal. For the other two the significance is based on a chi-squared test.

[2] In two weeks before each monthly interview.

[3] AQOL = asthma-related quality of life. Lower scores indicate poorer quality.

The results show that, where there is ETS exposure, the children have significantly greater absences from school and days and nights with symptoms and significantly less symptom-free days. The authors also noted that effects of school-based provision of ICS (improvement in symptoms, AQOL and absenteeism) were only seen among children not exposed to ETS.

1.3. Description of the Studies – Canada

The Vancouver Study

In the first paper based on this study, Murray and Morrison (1986) assessed the effect of parental smoking in 94 children with a history of asthmatic wheezing. The children were aged from 7 to 17, with 65% male. Only two admitted to smoking. There were 24 whose mother smoked and 70 where the mother was a non-smoker, the two groups being similar on age, gender and various confounding variables. Children whose mothers smoked had, on average, a 47% higher asthma history severity score (p=0.001), a 13% lower FEV_1 (p=0.004), a 23% lower $FEF_{25-75\%}$ (p=0.005) and, in a subgroup of 41 children whose values were not influenced by recent bronchodilator medications or by respiratory infections, an almost five-fold greater responsiveness to histamine (p=0.002). FVC was not significantly related to maternal smoking in all 94 children, but in the subgroup of 41 it was 12.6% lower (p=0.002) if the mother smoked. In all 94 children and in the subgroup, there was a significant dose-response to the number of cigarettes smoked by the mother at home for FVC, FEV_1, $FEF_{25-75\%}$, symptoms and responsiveness to histamine. The differences between the children of smoking and non-smoking mothers were greater in older than in younger subjects. In contrast there was no significant relationship of father's smoking to any of these indices of asthma severity, there being 28 children whose father smoked.

In an increased sample from this study, Murray and Morrison (1988) studied the effect of parental smoking in 240 non-smoking children with a history of asthmatic wheezing. The children were of age 7 to 17, with 68% male. As in the previous paper (Murray and Morrison, 1986), the overall data showed a strong relationship of maternal smoking to pulmonary function and bronchial responsiveness (symptom data not being reported this time), but little relationship to paternal smoking. There were 56 children with a mother who smoked and 183 with a non-smoking mother. Apart from the size of mite test reaction being smaller if the mother smoked ($p<0.01$), there was little difference between the two groups in potential confounding variables. Children with a smoking mother had a lower FEV_1 (76% vs 85%, $p<0.01$), a lower $FEF_{25-75\%}$ (59% vs 73%, $p<0.01$) and a lower PC_{20} (0.91 vs 2.03, p=0.01). There was also a strong correlation with the number of cigarettes smoked by the mother. Smaller differences were seen in relation to father's smoking and they were not statistically significant.

An interesting feature of the study is the separate analyses conducted according to whether or not the readings were taken in the cold, wet season (October-May), when windows would tend to be closed and ETS exposure higher, or in the warm, dry season (July-September), when windows tend to be open and exposure lower. The analyses showed a clear association of maternal smoking with pulmonary function (FEV_1 and $FEF_{25-75\%}$), bronchial responsiveness (PC_{20}) and recent use of bronchodilator medication in the cold, wet season, but no such association in the warm, dry season. These results were confirmed by analyses adjusting for potential confounding variables.

A third paper from this study (Murray and Morrison, 1989) was based on 414 non-smoking asthmatic children aged 1 to 17 (70% male) who had a mother with known smoking status. Only children aged 6+ underwent lung function testing, 294 producing an acceptable spirogram. As in the previous paper (Murray and Morrison, 1988) children of non-smoking mothers (n=322) and of smoking mothers (n=92) were comparable apart from the latter group of children having a smaller mite test wheal. Children of smoking mothers had a significantly higher asthma symptom score (8.8 vs 6.4, $p<0.01$), lower FEV_1 (77.3% vs 84.4%, $p<0.01$) lower $FEF_{25-75\%}$ (59.5% vs 71.7%, $p<0.01$) and lower log PC_{20} (-0.14 vs 0.71, $p=0.01$) and a non-significantly lower FVC (91.2% vs 93.8%, $p=0.2$). Although the differences were in the same direction in relation to smoking by the father, they were not statistically significant at $p<0.05$.

The main purpose of this paper was to investigate how the association with maternal smoking varied by the sex and age of the child. Associations tended to be stronger in boys than in girls and stronger in older than younger children. Although on some occasions differences according to maternal smoking status were significant for boys and not girls or for older and not younger children, the authors never actually carried out statistical tests of interaction. Based on the data presented we find that none of the differences between smoking and non-smoking parents vary significantly by the sex of the child and only for PC_{20} does the difference clearly vary significantly by age. As a result of this, we believe that the authors may have rather over-interpreted their data when they concluded that *"compared with girls, boys were more sensitive to passive smoking, and that its adverse effect increased with age and with duration of exposure."*

A fourth paper from the study in Vancouver (Murray and Morrison, 1992) concerned 240 non-smoking asthmatic children aged 7 to 17. As reported previously (Murray and Morrison, 1986; Murray and Morrison, 1988; Murray and Morrison, 1989), children whose mothers smoked had significantly more severe asthma. Since the children analysed in this paper are a subset of those described in the third paper (Murray and Morrison, 1989), the results add little new. The purpose of the paper was to investigate the effect of maternal smoking on asthma severity separately for those children who did or did not have atopic dermatitis, the analyses concluding that atopic dermatitis had no effect on asthma severity and that there was no interaction of atopic dermatitis with maternal smoking on severity.

The final paper from the study (Murray and Morrison, 1993) concerned 807 non-smoking children with asthma aged 1-17 years referred between 1983 and 1990. Comparisons were made of the 415 children seen before July 1986, and the 392 children seen afterwards. Doctors referring patients to the clinic have, since 1985, been urged to counsel parents of asthmatic children never to smoke when in the home. The main findings of the study were as follows:

- Although the total number of cigarettes smoked per day by parents was similar for the two periods, there was a highly significant drop in the number of cigarettes reported to be smoked in the presence of the child, from 7 to 3 for the mother, and from 5 to 2 for the father.
- Where the mother was a smoker, there was a highly significant ($p<0.001$) decline in the asthma score and increase in FEV_1 and $FEF_{25\text{-}75\%}$ between the two periods. In contrast, where the mother was a non-smoker, there was no decline in asthma score, and a smaller increase in lung function. A similar pattern was seen in relation to paternal smoking except that the decline in asthma score was not significant.
- The number of cigarettes reported to be smoked in the presence of the child by the mother was significantly correlated with the child's asthma score (positive) and with the two indices of lung function (negative). Similar correlations with paternal smoking were also significant for lung function but not for asthma score.
- Adjustment for sex, age, and age of onset of asthma confirmed the relationships noted in bullet point 2 above. Further adjustment for number of cigarettes smoked by the parents when in the same room as the child reduced the significance of the association.

The authors concluded that *"there is evidence that since 1986 an increasing awareness of the harmful effects of second-hand smoke has caused parents to smoke fewer cigarettes when with their asthmatic children, and that the resulting decrease in exposure has been associated with a marked improvement in the severity of asthma of the smokers' children who have been referred to our clinic."*

In considering these results, some important points should be made. Firstly, smoking habits of the parents were usually provided only by the mother and were unvalidated. It seems possible that at least part of the reported reduction in smoking in the presence of the child by the parents may have resulted from increasing denial. After all, there is abundant evidence in the literature that people advised by their doctor to give up smoking frequently falsely admit that they have done so (Lee, 1988). A similar scenario seems likely to exist if, as here, the doctor advised parents not to smoke in the presence of the child.

Second, the study showed no real evidence at all that bronchial hyper-responsiveness, as measured by the PC_{20} test, was associated with smoking by the parents or that it decreased between the two periods.

Third, on inspecting the detailed results presented, a striking fact emerges, namely that though in the first period the mean asthma score was highly significantly ($p<0.001$) *higher* if the mother smoked (mean 8.2, SE 0.3) than if the mother did not smoke (mean 6.4, SE 0.2), in the second period the mean asthma score was actually significantly ($p<0.05$) *lower* if the mother smoked (mean 5.8, SE 0.2) than if the mother did not smoke (mean 6.6, SE 0.2). The authors failed to mention this point, which seems inconsistent with their thesis. It is also true that, while before July 1986 pulmonary function was much lower if the mother smoked, after July 1986 it was very similar in children whose mothers smoked or did not smoke.

Finally, and importantly, one can compute from the results presented the following differences between the two time periods for children where the parent smokes:

	Difference post- vs pre-July 1986	
	Unadjusted[1]	Adjusted[1]
Asthma score	-0.99	-1.02
FEV_1%	+14.5	+11.4
$FEF_{25-75\%}$	+14.7	+11.95

[1] For number of cigarettes smoked in same room as child.

It can be seen that only a small proportion of the difference in recorded response between the two time periods (and essentially none of it as regards asthma score) can be explained by the parents smoking less in front of their children. This is in direct contrast to the authors' claims. Although there has been a marked improvement in asthma score and lung function over the period in children of smokers, it appears to be mainly due to reasons other than reduced smoking by the parents in the child's presence. It is also notable from the data presented in the paper that there were quite substantial improvements in lung function (though not in asthma score) over the time period in children whose parents do not smoke.

Generally, the paper must be regarded as unconvincing, with parts of the data inconsistent with the authors' claims not really brought to the reader's attention.

The Toronto Study

MacArthur et al. (1996) studied 68 children of median age 3 years, 71% male, who had their first ever admission for treatment of asthma in a defined 19 month period and who had been readmitted to the same hospital because of asthma within 12 months of the first admission. This cohort was followed forward, and their probability of readmission within 12 months of the second discharge related to a variety of risk factors. 17 of the 30 (57%) subjects with one or more smokers in the home qualified in this respect, as against 15 of the 38 (39%) with no smokers in the home. This represented a non-significant relative risk of 1.44 (95% CI 0.87-2.37).

The Edmonton Study

Mayo (2001) compared 31 children of mean age 6.4 years, 17 male, who had been admitted to a pediatric unit with an acute exacerbation of asthma of non-infectious origin and who had one or more parents who smoked at least a pack a day with 31 age- and sex-matched controls also with an acute exacerbation of asthma, but without such ETS exposure. Though the study principally concerned theophylline clearance, it was noted that the duration of the hospital stay was significantly ($p<0.05$) longer in the ETS-exposed group (4.35 vs 2.86 days). The author concluded that *"Clinically, passive smoke exposure resulted in a longer hospital stay"* without discussion or consideration of potential bias and confounding.

The Nine Region Study

A study in nine health units/departments across Canada (Dales et al., 2002) involved 3010 schoolchildren aged 5-19 years with current asthma, 52% of whom were male. The OR for having a hospital visit for asthma in the last 12 months in relation to regular ETS exposure at home was 1.55 (95% CI 1.22-1.97) in unadjusted analyses. The OR was noted to vary by household income (<$20000 1.79, $20000 to $60000 1.35, >$60000 1.45) although this variation did not appear to be statistically significant.

1.4. Description of the Studies – Europe

England: The Sheffield Study

In a case-control study, Strachan and Carey (1995) compared 486 secondary-school children who, in an earlier study two years before, had reported that over the previous 12 months they had suffered either 12 or more wheezing attacks or a speech-limiting attack of wheeze (over 90% of whom had doctor-diagnosed asthma) to 475 children with no history of asthma or wheeze, frequency matched for age and school class. While comparison of cases and controls is not relevant to exacerbation of asthma, tables are presented which allow comparison of parental smoking habits among 113 children with frequent and speech-limiting wheeze ("severe cases") and children with frequent or speech-limiting wheeze but not both ("less severe cases"). As shown in the table below, there was a significant tendency for severity of asthma to be greater if either the mother or the father smoked. However no dose-relationship was evident. The authors reported that results were similar for maternal smoking around the time of the child's birth, but did not present any details.

		Smoking habits (cigs/day)			
Parent	Asthma	0	1-10	>10	Any
Mother	Less severe	289	57	27	84
	Severe	75	25	13	38
	OR	1.00	1.69	1.86	1.74
	(95% CI)		(0.99-2.88)	(0.91-3.77)	(1.10-2.76)
Father	Less severe	313	39	20	59
	Severe	85	18	9	27
	OR	1.00	1.70	1.66	1.69
	(95% CI)		(0.93-3.12)	(0.73-3.77)	(1.01-2.82)

England: The North East England Study

Shamssain and Shamsian (1999) collected data on 3000 children aged 6-7 years from parents or guardians on smoking habits and on prevalence of various respiratory symptoms. About 685 children (59% male) had ever had asthma. The prevalence of ever asthma in the children was 20.6% if no parent smoked, 26.4% if one parent smoked and 28.7% if both parents smoked. Corresponding prevalences of limitation of speech during attacks in the past year were 2.7%,

3.7% and 4.3%. This implies that, among the asthmatics, the corresponding proportions with speech limitation were 13.1%, 14.0% and 15.0%, differences which are clearly not significant.

Finland: The Kuopio Study

Schwartz et al. (2000) studied 74 asthmatic children aged 7-12, 61% male. For three months the children measured their PEFR every morning and evening and kept a daily diary of respiratory symptoms. They also noted daily whether they had used respiratory medication and whether someone had smoked inside their home. When the data were analysed longitudinally, ETS exposure at home was associated with significant reductions in morning PEFR of 41.9 ℓ/min (95% CI 9.5 to 74.3 ℓ/min) and in evening PEFR of 40.7 ℓ/min (7.6 to 73.7 ℓ/min) after adjustment for age, height, sex, atopic status, father's education, weight, use of maintenance drugs, day of study, previous day's temperature and humidity, bronchodilator use, a random-subject effect, and whether the measurement was taken on a weekend. Similar estimates were obtained using a cross-sectional model. Adjustment for atopic status, use of maintenance drugs or bronchodilator use made little difference to the estimates, but failure to adjust for father's educational level would have led to markedly lower estimates of 26.0 ℓ/min for morning PEFR and of 23.8 ℓ/min for evening PEFR. Evidence was also presented to support the existence of a dose-related relationship (trend p=0.01) between PEFR and the percentage of days with ETS exposure. The above analyses were based on between-child comparisons. Within-child comparisons showed that ETS exposure on a given day was on average associated non-significantly with a lower PEFR the next day by about 10 ℓ/min.

The previous day's ETS exposure was a significant risk factor for need for bronchodilator use on any given day (OR 10.3, 95% CI 1.3-83.7). Mean ETS exposure over the previous two days was associated with a significant increase in the probability of cough (12.4, 2.4-63.3) and of phlegm production (7.8, 1.4-41.7). Wheezing/breathing difficulties were too rare for analysis.

The authors concluded *that "exposure to ETS was associated with a decline in peak flow and increase in symptom reporting and use of bronchodilator drugs by asthmatic children. The effect of ETS on PEFR in this study was largely chronic, but evidence for an effect of daily variations in ETS was seen for bronchodilator use and respiratory symptoms, and there was a suggestion of an acute effect on PEFR."*

France: The Marseilles Study

Dubus et al. (1998) studied 46 asthmatic children with a positive skin prick test (SPT) to one or more common aeroallergens, normal spirometric values and no upper airway infection. The children were aged 5 to 14 (mean 8.3), with 57% male. Parents were instructed to withhold any asthma therapy for 24h before the tests. Comparisons were made between 23 children with detectable and 23 with non-detectable cotinine in urine, based on a limit of detection of 1 ng/ml. No child was considered an active smoker based on the cotinine values (maximum = 98 ng/ml). There was no significant difference between the exposed (detectable cotinine) and unexposed groups in respect of the number of crises per year (4.1 vs 4.4), symptoms between crises (OR 0.49, CI 0.15-1.60) or use of anti-inflammatory treatment (0.66, 0.19-2.35). There was also no significant difference as regards FEV_1 (106.5% vs 101.9%, p=0.2), FVC (106.6% vs 101.7%, p=0.13), PEFR (89.1% vs 85.6%, p=0.56), $FEF_{25-75\%}$ (94.0% vs 104.3%, p=0.34), or SRAW (7.6 vs 7.4 cm H_2O/s, p=0.30). The doubling dose (PC_{100} SRAW) was determined, and was significantly less in the exposed group (108.3 vs 160.9 µg, p=0.04). Following administration of 200 µg albuterol, the percentage of bronchodilatation was defined from the difference between the largest SRAW value obtained and the SRAW value measured 15 minutes later divided by the largest SRAW value. This was significantly higher in the exposed group (74.8% vs 68.8%, p=0.03). No significant relationship was reported between parental smoking and either the doubling dose (mother smoked 98.4 vs 147.2 µg) or the percentage of bronchodilation (data not given). The authors concluded that *"environmental tobacco smoke increases bronchial reactivity in asthmatic and allergic children."*

A further report from Marseilles (Oddoze et al., 1999) concerned 90 children with suspected asthma, aged 4 to 14 (mean 8), with 60% male. The authors noted that urinary cotinine was not associated with basal spirometric tests (FEV_1 and SRAW). Bronchial responsiveness to carbachol was significantly associated with cotinine (p=0.03), but not CCR (p=0.07) or the number of cigarettes smoked by the parents (p=0.19). Detailed results were not reported. Despite these rather marginal results, the lack of consideration of any potential confounding variables and the fact that only 33% of the children had clinical asthma, the authors concluded that *"Passive smoke exposure increases the bronchial responsiveness to carbachol in asthmatic children."* Whether the samples of children studied in this and the previous paper are separate is unclear.

France: The Nationwide Study

A prospective study conducted by chest specialists throughout France (Soussan et al., 2003) involved 167 children aged 6-12 years (64% boys) with recently diagnosed mild or moderate persistent asthma who had been prescribed inhaled anti-inflammatory treatment. Starting one year after recruitment, the children were followed-up for a further 2 years, with a visit every 4 months. PEF was measured twice a day during the week before each visit. Two endpoints were studied: (1) symptom control = having diurnal or nocturnal exacerbations less than once a week and no symptoms between exacerbations, at all visits and (2) PEF control = daily PEF variability <20% on each of the seven days before each visit. Symptom control was achieved by 42 children and PEF control by 89. 28 factors were considered, of which 10, including the ETS variable at least one smoker in the home, were related to symptom control in univariate analysis (p<0.2) and were included in a multiple regression analysis. Three factors remained significantly (p<0.05) related to symptom control – taking the prescribed doses (OR = 4.82, 95% CI = 1.87-12.4), understanding how the medication works (3.38, 1.18-9.64) and at least one smoker in the home (0.34, 0.13-0.91). Similarly, of 9 factors, including the ETS variable mother smoking in the home, identified in the univariate analysis for PEF control, taking the prescribed doses (3.58, 1.68-7.67), moulds within the home (0.33, 0.11-0.97) and mother smoking in the home (0.34, 0.14-0.89) remained significant in the multivariate analysis. Although taking the prescribed doses was a major factor for both endpoints, no information was presented on whether children with smokers in the home were more or less likely to take the prescribed doses (or understand how the medication works). It should be noted that the endpoints can be seen as inversely related to asthma severity/exacerbation.

Germany: The Freiburg Study

Frischer et al. (1992) investigated the relationship between maternal smoking and bronchial hyperresponsiveness (as assessed by a decrease of 15% or greater in PEFR following a standardized free running test) in 1461 primary school children of mean age 7.3 years. 171 of the children were asthmatics. Among this group the prevalence of bronchial hyperresponsiveness was non-significantly higher if the mother smoked in pregnancy (22.2% vs 14.5%) or if the mother smoked in the child's first year (24.2% vs 13.5%), but was non-significantly lower if the mother smoked in the child's eight year (9.5% vs 17.7%). In a multivariate analysis involving prematurity, pneumonia during the first year of life, atopy, education and sex of the child, the authors reported no significant relationship to maternal smoking in pregnancy (OR 2.20, 95% CI 0.29-16.57), a significant and huge positive relationship to maternal smoking in the child's first year (20.56, 2.5-168.9) and a significant and huge negative relationship to maternal smoking in the child's eight year (0.05, 0.005-0.61). It seems to us that these analyses may be unstable due to the strong correlations between maternal smoking at the various time points, and that the association of ETS with bronchial hyperresponsiveness is unclear from these data. However, the authors cited the findings in the abstract, noting the very strong positive OR with maternal smoking in the child's first year, but also noting that *"current exposure to maternal smoking was associated with less hyperresponsiveness."* They commented that *"The effect of current maternal smoking might reflect changes in smoking habits by mothers of children with symptoms, whereas exposure to tobacco smoke in early life might be causally related to bronchial hyperresponsiveness,"* and concluded by stating that *"Our findings support the general hypothesis that early lung injuries have an impact on the later respiratory health of children."*

Meinert et al. (1994) presented essentially the same findings two years later, though the results, with ORs of 1.3 for mother smoked before pregnancy, 1.7 for smoking during pregnancy, 2.2 for smoking in the child's first year and 0.5 for smoking in the child's eighth year, were based on separate analyses. The authors reported a significant (p=0.02) association between bronchial hyperresponsiveness and changes in maternal smoking habits between the child's first and eight years.

Change in smoking habit	% of children with BHR	% of children without BHR
Began smoking after pregnancy	20	8
Began smoking between 1st and 8th year	0	12
Stopped smoking between 1st and 8th year	16	3

BHR = bronchial hyperresponsiveness.

Based on the same study, Frischer et al. (1993) reported the relationship of maternal and paternal smoking to PEFR variability based on 991 of the 7 year old children (48% male), 113 of whom were asthmatic. The PEFR was measured twice daily over a 1 week period, with the log of a week's mean of daily amplitude calculated as an index of variability. In multivariate analysis, only current maternal smoking and atopy were found to have a significant relationship to PEFR variability. For asthmatic children without atopy (n=80), PEFR variability was 54.7% higher (95% CI +5.5% to +226.8%) if the mother smoked, whereas in atopic asthmatic children (n=33), it was 8.5% lower (95% CI –41.2% to +42.3%). In the latter group there was evidence that mothers changed their smoking habits subsequent to the development of disease in their children. The authors concluded that *"exposure to maternal smoking can increase the variability of PEFR and thus might contribute to the development of asthma."*

Germany: The Lower Saxony Study

Seidler et al. (1998) studied 600 asthmatic children aged up to 8 years who had attended a doctor in a baseline phase in 1991. 218 (65% male) of the children had visited the same doctor about 3 years later during a follow-up phase. There were 200 children with information on progression of the asthma; 29% with no attacks, 45% with a decreasing frequency of attacks over the 3 years, 20% in which the frequency had remained the same and 7% in which it had increased. In a polytomous logistic regression analysis involving a number of other variables (age, sex, parental education, frequency of asthmatic episodes, infection-associated asthma, "asthma on exertion," neurodermitis of the child, hospital stay, speciality of treating physician, adequacy of medication, parental asthma, sensitivity to exhaust gases and region) smoking in the home was associated with a marginally significant (p=0.05) increased risk of an unfavourable course of the disease, with an OR of 1.7 (95% CI 1.0-3.0). It is not totally clear to these reviewers whether all variables were considered simultaneously in the analysis or whether Table 3 of the source paper presents the results of univariate analysis. As a multivariate analysis it would have some objections in that asthma endpoints seem to be included both as independent and dependent variables. An association was reported between having more than five asthmatic episodes in the last 12 months and a worsening course of the disease, but these variables to some extent measure the same thing. The authors did not include any simple table relating smoking in the home to progression of the asthma. The paper also reported an almost significant (0.05<p<0.1) difference in the prevalence of smoking in the home for the 382 children not followed up (42%) and the 218 followed up (34%). This highlights the possibility of some selection bias.

Italy: The Viterbo Province Study

Martinez et al. (1988) studied the relationship between parental smoking, asthmatic status, atopy and bronchial responsiveness in 170 unselected schoolchildren aged 9, 49% of whom were boys. The relationship of bronchial responsiveness (as determined by a carbachol inhalation test to obtain a drop in FEV_1 of 20% or more) to parental smoking in the whole population was significant (p=0.036) after controlling for sex and atopy. In the 22 asthmatic children, the same relationship was significantly (p=0.02) stronger, with the OR for bronchial responsiveness for parental smoking estimated as 18.7 (1.5-232.3), based on 14/17 responders where a parent smoked and 1/5 responders where no parent smoked.

Netherlands: The Zwolle Study

Meijer et al. (1996) studied 55 children of mean age 9.3 years, 60% boys, who had symptoms of asthma, increased total IgE, an allergy to house dust mite (HDM) but not to dog, cat, tree, grass or milk, an $FEV_1 \geq 70\%$ of the predicted value and increased bronchial responsiveness to histamine. The children all had asthma symptoms well controlled by daily ICS and β_2-adrenergic drugs if needed. PEFR amplitude (mean % over a 24 hour period) was obtained during and 6 days after withdrawal of ICS. 26 of the 55 children had a parent who smoked. PEFR amplitude in relation to ETS (from parental smoking) and ICS withdrawal was as follows:

		Median (Minimum-Maximum) PEFR amplitude	
Exposure	n	During ICS	After ICS withdrawal
No ETS	29	20.6 (5.7-63.4)	19.4 (0.0-56.5)
ETS	26	28.7 (10.7-99.0)	29.7 (3.9-56.6)
Significance of difference[1]		Not significant (p>0.05)	p<0.05

[1] From Mann-Whitney U test.

The authors noted that *"children exposed to ETS ... had significantly higher PEFR amplitudes after withdrawal of ICS than did nonexposed children"* and that *"This was not found during ICS"* and concluded that *"exogenous stimuli such as exposure to ETS ... contribute to an increased circadian PEFR amplitude after withdrawal of ICS and therefore to nocturnal worsening of asthma in HDM-*

allergic asthmatic children." But the difference in medians between ETS and non-ETS exposed children is in fact very similar during ICS (28.7-20.6 = 8.1) and after ICS withdrawal (29.7-19.4 = 10.3) and is clearly not significantly different.

The authors also reported the results of a multivariate analysis investigating factors associated with PEFR amplitude after withdrawal of ICS. Although the difference associated with ETS increased only slightly, from 10.3 to 11.2, the p value now became highly significant ($p<0.001$). The authors also noted an interaction between the effects of ETS and of bronchial responsiveness on PEFR amplitude after ICS withdrawal, finding a significant association between ETS and PEFR amplitude only in those with an above average bronchial responsiveness ($p=0.008$). Given that the difference in amplitude associated with ETS exposure is only significant at $p=0.05$ for those with above average responsiveness, and that the difference is in the same direction for those with below average responsiveness, it is difficult to see how the interaction is in fact significant at all, let alone significant at $p=0.008$.

Apart from these doubts about the validity of the statistical analysis, one must also wonder how the endpoint of the study, PEFR amplitude, actually relates to exacerbation of asthma. It should be noted that their own data showed no relationship of FEV_1 to PEFR amplitude.

Portugal: The Lisbon Study

Gaspar et al. (2002) compared 124 children admitted to a hospital for acute asthma during a two-year period (mean age 4.1 years, 57% male) to 124 outpatients individually matched on age, sex and socio-economic status. In univariate analyses asthma admission was significantly associated with parental smoking (OR 3.51, 95% CI 2.1-6.0), paternal smoking (3.0, 1.8-4.9), maternal smoking (1.8, 1.0-3.1, $p=0.02$) and with any ETS exposure (4.59, 2.6-8.0), but not with other residents at the home (1.28, 0.8-2.0). Similar relationships were seen when analysis was restricted to the 74 pairs of children under 4 years of age – e.g. for any ETS exposure (5.0, 2.3-11.4). In a multiple logistic regression analysis involving all the children, any ETS exposure remained a significant predictor of asthma admission (6.63, 2.5-17.8) after adjustment for prior asthma hospitalisation, atopy, maternal asthma, last year asthma admission, onset of symptoms before 12 months of age, attendance at day care or kindergarten, and family size.

Scotland: The Tayside and Fife Study

Crombie et al. (2001) studied 438 asthmatic children aged 2-12, 66% of whom were male and all having one or more parents who smoked. They had previously taken part in a randomised controlled trial of advice aimed at reducing passive smoking. Information on health service contacts for asthma over the previous 12 months was collected and a saliva sample taken for cotinine determination. In a multivariate model including age, severity of asthma (perceived, and based on treatment) and number of children in the household, there was no clear relationship of cotinine to the frequency of contacts for asthma, with incidence rate ratios of 0.95 (95% CI 0.82-1.11) for medium cotinine (2.1-4.5 ng/ml) and of 1.15 (0.98-1.34) for high cotinine (>4.5 ng/ml) as compared to low cotinine (≤2.0 ng/ml). In the same model, there was a significant tendency for the incidence rate ratio to be reduced if the mother only smoked (0.76, 0.64-0.89) or if both parents smoked (0.78, 0.66-0.93) compared to if the father only smoked. In earlier univariate analysis, the authors had also reported a highly significant negative relationship with the amount smoked in the home by the index parent, with incidence ratios of 1.00, 0.81, 0.70, 0.74 and 0.66 for, respectively, 0-5, 6-10, 11-15, 16-20 and >20 cigarettes/day, although amount smoked in the home did not appear in the final multivariate model. The authors concluded that *"High levels of parental smoking in the home are associated with a reduction in health care contacts for asthma. This could be due to a lack of awareness of asthma symptoms among heavy smokers or a reluctance to visit the GP. Children with asthma who have parents who smoke heavily may not be receiving adequate management."* [GP is general practitioner.]

Spain: The San Sebastian Study

Callén et al. (1997) studied 312 asthmatic children aged 3-19 years (mean 9.01), comparing 187 cases satisfying at least one of the following criteria: FVC < 85%, FEV_1 < 85%, PEFR < 85% or $FEF_{25\text{-}75\%}$ < 60%, and 125 controls satisfying none of these. One or more parents smoked in 70.1% of the cases and 56.0% of the controls, giving an OR of 1.84 (95% CI 1.12-3.03). The authors also presented a table comparing pulmonary function variables according to at home ETS exposure, presumably based on all 312 children. For all four variables, values were lower in the exposed group (FVC 96.9% vs 97.4%, FEV_1 91.9% vs 93.7%, PEFR 87.2% vs 92.6%, $FEF_{25\text{-}75\%}$ 72.2% vs 76.7%) but none of the differences were statistically significant, with the p values >0.2 for each comparison. Despite this lack of association, one of the conclusions was that *"pulmonary function in asthmatic children is influenced by parental smoking habits."* The basis for this conclusion is not apparent. COHb was measured in both children and parents. Though results were presented which found that smoking parents had higher COHb, it seems somewhat surprising that the child's COHb was not compared in the two groups of asthmatic children.

Sweden: The Stockholm Study

In an abstract describing a two-year follow-up of a study of asthmatic children Melén et al. (2000) reported results for 144 of the original 189 children. 12 children of mean age 44.3 months were assessed as having severe asthma (based on symptoms and use of inhaled steroids) and 132 children of mean age 49.5 months were assessed as having mild/moderate asthma. Parental smoking was one of a number of variables recorded at baseline (age 1-4) associated with an increased risk of severe asthma at follow-up (age 3-6), with a relative risk estimated as 2.7 (95% CI 0.8-9.8). Parental smoking at follow-up was also stated to have no significant association. It was not stated whether these analyses were adjusted for potential confounding factors. Although the relative risks for parental smoking were not statistically significant the authors nevertheless concluded that *"In children with induction of asthma during the first two years of life, early sensitization, cat allergen exposure at home and parental smoking seem to increase the risk for development of severe asthma with regular use of inhaled steroids later in childhood."*

Later Melén et al. (2001) reported results based on 181 asthmatic children aged 1-4, 76% male, who were followed up for 2 years. Of 12 children satisfying the criteria for current severe asthma at follow-up, 9 (75%) had reported ETS exposure at home at baseline whereas, of 158 children with mild/moderate asthma, 85 (54%) did. This was reported as a non-significant OR of 2.59 (95% CI 0.73-9.14) [though from the data presented we calculate it as 2.58 (0.67-9.87)]. After adjustment for age, heredity, and exposure to cat, dog and windowpane condensation, the OR increased to 3.01 (0.74-12.2) but remained non-significant. The unadjusted OR is equivalent to a relative risk of 1.39 (0.61-3.18). The number of children with severe asthma is too small to make any firm conclusion, though the authors noted that *"In young asthmatic children, early exposure to ... tobacco smoke increased the risk of ... further development of more severe asthma later in childhood."* The subjects in this study possibly include those described in the earlier abstract.

1.5. Description of the Studies – Asia (Including Turkey)

China: The Anqing Study

Venners et al. (2001) studied 529 never smoking asthmatic children aged 8 to 15 years of age whose mother was a never smoker. 50% of the children were male. As shown in the table below, both in girls and boys, paternal smoking was associated with some reduction in FEV_1 and FVC after adjustment for age, height, height squared, weight and father's education. However these relationships were not statistically significant.

		Decrement in FEV_1 or FVC by father's smoking habits[1]		
Endpoint	Sex	Never	<30 cigs/day	30+ cigs/day
FEV_1	Boys	0 (base)	-1.9%	-3.7%
	Girls	0	-1.0%	-1.3%
FVC	Boys	0	-1.8%	-3.7%
	Girls	0	-0.4%	-0.8%
		Number of subjects		
	Boys	48	179	38
	Girls	50	185	29

[1] Ex-smoking fathers were excluded.

The authors stated that they also investigated the ratio of FEV_1 to FVC but did not find an important association.

India: The New Delhi Study

Ratageri et al. (2000) studied 60 children suffering from severe chronic asthma and 60 children suffering from mild chronic asthma. The children were aged 5-15 years with 72% male. On univariate analysis there was a tendency for the odds of severe asthma to be increased if family members smoked, particularly 10+ cigs/day. In multivariate analysis involving age of onset of asthma, past history of lung diseases, family history of asthma, allergy, breastfeeding, overcrowding, pets, cooking, worm infestation, eosinophil count and air pollution, smoking by the family did not emerge as a factor associated with severity of asthma.

	Mild		Severe		
Smoking by the family	No	Yes	No	Yes	OR (95% CI)
Any family member	32	28	26	34	1.49 (0.73-3.07)
Father	38	22	31	29	1.62 (0.78-3.35)
Grandfather	55	5	54	6	1.22 (0.35-4.24)
Cigs/day smoked by family:					
None		23		26	1.00
1-9		13		7	0.66 (0.23-1.90)
10		15		27	2.22 (0.98-5.01)

Lebanon: The Tripoli Study

A retrospective study (Kalaajieh, 2002) involved 288 asthmatic children between 6 and 15 years of age, 64% male, who were hospitalised over an 8 year period. Data on ETS exposure at birth and other factors were recorded at the time of first admission and related to the rate of further admissions by the end of the period. 68 of the children had a mean of more than one further admission per year. In univariate analyses, 13 factors were identified as having a significant association with multiple admission. These included maternal smoking (OR 6.10, 95% CI 2.98-12.55) and indoor smoking (3.06, 1.81-5.18), and also sex, age, residence, frequent respiratory tract infection, atopic dermatitis, allergic conjunctivitis, allergic rhinitis, family history of allergy, total serum IgE, eosinophils in peripheral blood and household number. Although many of these associations were very strong and highly significant (e.g. atopic dermatitis 11.93, 5.81-24.53), only two factors were found to be significant in a multiple logistic regression analysis – maternal smoking and recurrent URI (both $p<0.001$; ORs not given).

Saudi Arabia: The Al-Majmaah Study

Al-Ghamdy et al. (2000) studied 606 children with asthma aged up to 13 years, 69% male. 292 of these were infants aged less than 1 year. The authors presented a table relating asthma severity (based on national guidelines) to parental smoking from which the relative risks given below were calculated and showed a significant relationship. No attempt was made to adjust for potential confounding factors.

Parental smoking	Asthma severity		
	Mild	Moderate	Severe
No	279	30	29
Yes	190	37	41
OR	1.00	1.81	2.08
(95% CI)		(1.08-3.03)	(1.25-3.46)

Taiwan Study

In a study of 46 asthmatic children reported only as an abstract (Chan and Chen, 1995) peak expiratory flows (PEFRs) were measured at night and in the morning daily over a 6 month period, a PEFR lower than 80% of predicted being defined as an asthmatic attack. The CCR of urine samples collected at different PEFR levels was used as a biomarker for ETS exposure. The CCR associated with a PEFR ratio <0.8 was stated to be significantly higher than that associated with a PEFR ratio >0.8 (13.95 vs 7.09 ng/mg) for urine samples collected in the night, though the actual significance level was not given. There was also a significant trend in CCR increase as the PEFR ratio decreased. The abstract does not make clear how the multiple data per subject have been dealt with, and whether the analyses have been based on within- or between-subject comparisons. The data clearly have the potential to test whether, within-subject, PEFR varies by CCR, which would be valuable to know.

Turkey: The First Istanbul Study

A study reported only as an abstract (Güler et al., 2000) involved 47 asthmatic schoolchildren aged 5 to 15 years, with 68% boys. A questionnaire determined the amount and time of exposure to ETS, and the urinary CCR was determined. The patients were followed up for one year and pulmonary function was determined regularly. The abstract states that there was no correlation of asthma severity or pulmonary function to CCR. Asthma severity was, however, significantly correlated with the number of cigarettes smoked by the mother currently (p=0.008), by the mother during pregnancy (p=0.006), and by the father (p=0.04) and with the amount of passive smoking of mothers during pregnancy (p=0.04). $FEF_{25-75\%}$ reversibility (undefined) was significantly higher if the mother smoked currently (p=0.03) and during pregnancy (p=0.001). PEF reversibility (not defined) was significantly higher if the mother smoked during pregnancy (p not given). The authors considered that they *"have established that ETS, primarily smoked by the mother during various periods of life have (sic) long term effects on clinical features of asthma in schoolchildren."* They did not comment on the inferences to be drawn from the fact that an objective indicator of ETS exposure (CCR) found no association with asthma severity or pulmonary function but self-reported indicators did. It is unclear from the abstract which of the multiple pulmonary function measurements were used in the analysis. There was also no attempt to separate results for pre- and post-natal smoking.

Turkey: The Second Istanbul Study

Karadag et al. (2003) studied 32 children admitted to an emergency clinic with an acute asthma attack, 62.5% male. They ranged in age from 1 to 14 (mean 5.7 years). Urinary cotinine and creatinine levels were measured during and 4 weeks after the acute asthma attack. Comparing the period of the acute attack and the asymptomatic period, there was no significant difference in cotinine (295 vs 230 ng/ml), CCR (315 vs 204 ng/mg) or having a CCR above 30 ng/mg (81% vs 96%). It is not clear that the data from this study have been analysed correctly. It appears from the way the results are presented and the lack of reference to appropriate statistical tests that the analyses have been carried out as if two independent groups of 32 children are being compared, when tests should have been based on the distribution of within-subject differences, e.g. using a paired t-test. Whether this would have altered the significance of the difference between the time periods cannot be assessed.

Turkey: The Diyarbakir Study

Gürkan et al. (2000) studied hospital admissions retrospectively over a period of up to 4 years in 140 children with asthma aged 3-15 years, 65% male. Over the follow-up period 30 of the children (21.4%) had a mean of more than one admission per year and qualified as a multiple admission. Results relating multiple admissions to a range of factors were presented on an individual basis. These showed significant associations with both maternal smoking and smoking in the house, as summarized below:

		Multiple admissions		OR
		Yes	No	(95% CI)
Smoker in the house	Yes	16	34	2.55
	No	14	76	(1.12-5.82)
Maternal smoking	Yes	7	8	3.88[1]
	No	23	102	(1.28-11.8)

[1] Miscalculated as 4.05 (1.47-11.78) by the authors.

The authors also summarized the results of a multivariate logistic regression analysis in which only maternal smoking and age of the child were significant. They cited an adjusted OR of 3.25 (95% CI 1.13-8.85) for maternal smoking.

1.6. Description of the Studies – Other Areas

Kenya: The Nairobi Study

Wafula et al. (1999) studied 150 children with a history of wheezing with a mean age of 4 years (1 month - 10 years) with 60% male. The children were classified as having mild (32%), moderate (47%) or severe (21%) asthma, based on frequency of attacks. There was a non-significant tendency for passive smoke exposure at home to be associated with moderate asthma. Thus 36/71 children (51%) with moderate asthma were exposed to ETS as against 16/48 (33%) with mild asthma (OR 2.06, 95% CI 0.96-4.40). The definition of asthma used in this study required only *"at least two previous episodes of wheezing"* and seems very unrestrictive. It is also unexplained why passive smoking data were not presented for the severe cases. The only other risk factor considered in this study was breastfeeding and then not simultaneously with passive smoking.

New Zealand: The Christchurch Study

Fergusson and Horwood (1985) reported findings based on 1115 of an original 1265 children born in mid-1977 followed up to age 6 years. The relationship between parental smoking and respiratory illnesses during this period was studied. The authors presented the joint relationship of maternal and paternal smoking among the whole population to ever having had an asthmatic episode and to the rate of asthmatic attacks per 100 children. 134 children had a diagnosis of asthma or wheezy bronchitis, while 141 had a maternal report of an asthmatic attack. From these data we have estimated the annual rates per asthmatic child, separately for medical consultations and for maternal reports. The results show no apparent trend with paternal smoking, but some with maternal smoking, though it is impossible to assess statistical significance from the data provided.

	Source of	Smoking (cigs/day)		
Exposure	information on asthma	0	1-10	11+
Mother	Medical consultation	0.80	0.53	0.96
	Maternal report	1.59	0.96	2.03
Father	Medical consultation	0.82	0.64	0.85
	Maternal report	1.55	1.60	1.46

(Note that these data have been estimated by dividing the rate of attack per 100 children aged 0-6 by six times the risk per 100 children of having at least one episode by the age of 6 years. Strictly the rates per asthmatic child should be estimated during the period the child was asthmatic, but this cannot be done from the data available. Parental smoking was assessed on eight occasions, but it is unclear how parents who changed their smoking habits have been categorized.)

Nigeria: The Ibadan Study

Aderele (1982) studied 380 asthmatic children aged between 10 months and 13 years, with 62% male. 107 of the children had severe asthma, 87 had moderate asthma and 186 had mild disease. None of the children were known to be smokers. From the data presented one can calculate the following relative risk estimates (95% CI) for severe and moderate asthma compared to mild asthma.

Smoking by household members	Mild	Moderate	Severe
No	143	64	74
Adult	43	23	33
RR (95% CI)	1.00	1.20 (0.67-2.15)	1.48 (0.87-2.53)
Father and older siblings	20	16	27
RR (95% CI)	1.00	1.79 (0.87-3.67)	2.61 (1.37-4.96)
Other smoking (not father/siblings)	23	7	6
RR (95% CI)	1.00	0.68 (0.28-1.67)	0.50 (0.20-1.29)
Total	186	87	107

The author noted the significance ($p<0.01$) of the trend in relation to severity where the fathers and older siblings smoked, but did not discuss the implied negative relationship with severity in other households where there was a smoker. There was no adjustment for any confounding factors although data were collected on a wide variety of variables. The author also noted that 80 (34%) of the 234 children aged 5 years and above admitted they usually coughed on passively inhaling cigarette smoke.

South Africa: The Cape Town Study

Ehrlich et al. (2001) studied 249 children with asthma aged 6-11, 52% male, all of whom claimed never to have tried cigarettes, who underwent a test of bronchial responsiveness to histamine (or salbutamol if their FEV_1 was less than 75% of normal). In a multivariate analysis involving atopic history, baseline FEV_1, previous recognition of asthma by the parent, symptom score and medical insurance, a non-significant negative relationship was found between whether the chid responded to the test and mother's daily cigarettes, with the OR estimated as 0.97 (95% CI 0.67-1.41) for 1-14 cigs/day and 0.62 (0.34-1.11) for 15+ cigs/day. No significant associations were also found between bronchial responsiveness and other indices of parental smoking (current smoking or smoking in the first year of life by either parent individually, maternal smoking in pregnancy, number of smokers in the home or CCR). Nor was CCR related to the asthma symptom score. Baseline FEV_1, adjusted for age, sex and height, was also related to a variety of indices of smoking habits. There was no association with CCR. As shown in the table below, where selected results have been presented, there was a significant reduction in FEV_1 if the mother currently smoked or if both parents smoked, but a non-significant increase if the mother had ever smoked or if the father currently smoked.

The authors noted that *"the findings do not support a mechanism whereby ETS exposure aggravates existing childhood asthma by increasing BHR. This association may be masked, however, by the degree to which mothers of asthmatic children adjust their smoking. The results are consistent with an adverse effect of maternal smoking on lung function in asthmatic children."*

Exposure to smokers	Mean FEV$_1$, ml		Mean difference, ml (95% CI)	
	Exposed	Unexposed		
Mother current	1409	1641	-232	(-461 to -2)
Mother ever	1526	1467	+59	(-107[1] to +225)
Mother in pregnancy	1464	1557	-93	(-296 to +110)
Father current	1561	1449	+112	(-78 to +302)
Mother and father	1385	1591	-150	(-286 to -131)[2]
Two or more in household	1455	1591	-137	(-366 to +92)

[1] Given as 107 in the source paper, but clearly erroneous and should be -107.

[2] There appears to be some error in the data presented for mother and father smoking. The estimate of -150 for the difference is not equal to the difference of the means (-206). Nor is it in the middle of the 95% CI. The width of the CI, 155, is also far too small given the SEs of 32 and 62 for the two means which imply a width almost twice this.

1.7. Summary of the Studies

Table 1 summarizes some details of the studies on ETS and asthma exacerbation in children. As noted earlier, there are a total of 60 publications, which together appear to relate to 47 studies, though in some cases this is not clear. The table is presented in chronological order of the first publication from the study. Later publications from a study are shown on the lines following the first publication, with the location and country columns left blank. Other data in the table (numbers of asthmatics, % male, age and "includes smokers") are shown for each of the multiple publications. In the distributions described below (which are study- rather than publication-based) the values used are those which are not given in parentheses. The value selected for a study is generally taken from the publication based on most asthmatic subjects or providing most information.

Publication date. The first study was published in 1974, with two studies published in 1980-1984, five in 1985-1989, five in 1990-1994, 12 in 1995-1999 and 22 in 2000-2004. The steeply increasing publication rate is evident.

Location. Twenty-two studies have been conducted in North America, 18 in the USA and four in Canada. Thirteen studies have been conducted in Europe in a total of 10 countries, with no more than two from any country. Three studies have been in Turkey, two in the Middle East, three in India or the Far East, three in Africa and one in New Zealand. In all, studies have been conducted in 22 different countries. This represents quite an extensive geographical coverage, though no studies have been reported from Central or South America.

Most of the studies have been conducted in specific cities or areas, though results have been reported for two nationwide studies in the USA and one in France. One study in Canada was based on nine regions.

Number of asthmatic subjects. Based on the publication that considered the largest number of asthmatic subjects, the smallest study involved only 17 asthmatic subjects, while the largest is the nine region study in Canada (Dales et al., 2002) involving 3010. The median study size is 167. The distribution of study size is as follows:

Study size	17-50	51-100	101-250	251-500	501-1000	1001-3010
Studies	8	7	18	6	7	1

Sex of subjects. All studies either included both sexes, or did not state the sex of the subjects. Generally, there were more boys than girls, with the percentage of boys up to 76% (Table 1). Exceptions were the studies in Baltimore (Morkjaroenpong et al., 2002) and Seattle (Abulhosn et al., 1997) with about 40% boys.

Age of subjects. Table 1 shows the age range of the subjects where available or, except for one study where no information on age was provided, the mean or median age. Of the 43 studies that provided age range data, the number of studies where the range covered specific ages is as follows:

Age	0	1	2	3	4	5	6	7	8	9
Studies	7	13	16	22	25	31	35	36	35	35
Age	10	11	12	13	14	15	16	17	18	19
Studies	33	31	28	23	19	16	11	8	5	3

It can be seen that age 7 was the most commonly studied, with over 30 of the 43 studies providing data for ages in the range 5 to 11. The number of studies including infants (aged 0-1) or young adults (aged 16-19) was considerably less. The mean number of ages covered by the studies was 10, so it is clear that the tendency was not to concentrate on a very limited age range, though some studies did.

Table 1. Some details of the exacerbation studies in children

Publication[1]	Location[2]	Country[2]	Number of asthmatics[3]	% male[3,4]	Age[3,5]	Includes smokers[3,6]
O'Connell and Logan, 1974	Minnesota	USA	35[7]	60	2-16	NK
Aderele, 1982	Ibadan	Nigeria	380	62	1-13	No
Gortmaker et al., 1982	Michigan and Massachu-setts	USA	217	NK	0-17	NK
Fergusson and Horwood, 1985	Christchurch	New Zealand	141[8]	NK	0-6	NK
Murray and Morrison, 1986	Vancouver	Canada	(94)	(65)	(7-17)	(2)
Murray and Morrison, 1988			(240)	(68)	(7-17)	(No)
Murray and Morrison, 1989			(414)	70	(1-17)	(No)
Murray and Morrison, 1992			(240)	(NK)	(7-17)	(No)
Murray and Morrison, 1993			807	(NK)	1-17	No
Evans et al., 1987	New York	USA	191	60	4-17	No
O'Connor et al., 1987	Boston	USA	21	62	5-9	No
Martinez et al., 1988	Viterbo	Italy	22	NK	9	NK
Weitzman et al., 1990b	Nationwide	USA	117	NK	0-5	NK
Weitzman et al., 1990a			(110)	63	(2-5)	(NK)
Lilienfeld et al., 1990*	New York	USA	(107)	(NK)	(3-14)	(NK)
Ehrlich et al., 1992			107	62	3-14	No
Frischer et al., 1992	Freiburg	Germany	171	NK	mn7.3	NK
Frischer et al., 1993			(113)	(NK)	(md7.3)	(NK)
Meinert et al., 1994			(162)	(NK)	(8)	(NK)
Salmun et al., 1992*	Portland	USA	(199)	(NK)	(0-13)	(NK)
Chilmonczyk et al., 1993			199	72	0-13	NK
Ogborn et al., 1994	Baltimore	USA	56	57	3-11	NK
Abulhosn et al., 1995*	Seattle	USA	(22)	(NK)	(2-9)	(NK)
Abulhosn et al., 1997			22	41	2-13	NK
Chan and Chen, 1995*	Taiwan	Taiwan	46	NK	NK	NK

Table 1. Some details of the exacerbation studies in children (Continued)

Publication[1]	Location[2]	Country[2]	Number of asthmatics[3]	% male[3,4]	Age[3,5]	Includes smokers[3,6]
LeSon and Gershwin, 1995	Davis	USA	300	55	5-12	NK
Strachan and Carey, 1995	Sheffield	England	486	NK	12-18	NK
MacArthur et al., 1996	Toronto	Canada	68	71	md3	NK
Meijer et al., 1996	Zwolle	Nether-lands	55	60	mn9.3	NK
Callén Blecua et al., 1997	San Sebastian	Spain	312	NK	3-19	1
Hu et al., 1997	Chicago	USA	167	51	10-11[9]	5%[10]
Seidler et al., 1998	Lower Saxony	Germany	200	65	0-8	NK
Dubus et al., 1998	Marseilles	France	(46)	(57)	(5-14)	No
Oddoze et al., 1999			90	60	4-14	(NK)
Shamssain and Shamsian, 1999	N.E.England	England	685[11]	59	6-7	NK
Wafula et al., 1999	Nairobi	Kenya	150	60	0-10	NK
Al-Ghamdy et al., 2000	Al-Majmaah	Saudi Arabia	606	69	<13[12]	NK
El-Dahr et al., 2000*	New Orleans	USA	17	56	6-16	No
Güler et al., 2000*	Istanbul	Turkey	47	68	5-15	NK
Gürkan et al., 2000	Diyarbakir	Turkey	140	65	3-15	NK
Li et al., 2000	S.California	USA	749	59	7-19	13
Melén et al., 2000*	Stockholm	Sweden	(144)	(NK)	(1-6)	(NK)
Melén et al., 2001			181	76	1-6	NK
Ratageri et al., 2000	New Delhi	India	120	72	5-15	NK
Schwartz et al., 2000	Kuopio	Finland	74	61	7-12	NK
Crombie et al., 2001	Tayside and Fife	Scotland	438	66	2-12	NK
Ehrlich et al., 2001	Cape Town	South Africa	249	52	6-11	No
Mayo, 2001	Edmonton	Canada	62	55	1-9	NK
Venners et al., 2001	Anqing	China	529	50	8-15	Never
Wilson et al., 2001b	California	USA	87	51	3-12	NK
Dales et al., 2002	9 regions	Canada	3010	52	5-19	NK
Gaspar et al., 2002	Lisbon	Portugal	248	57	1-10	NK
Kalaajieh, 2002	Tripoli	Lebanon	288	64	6-15	NK

Table 1. Some details of the exacerbation studies in children (Continued)

Publication[1]	Location[2]	Country[2]	Number of asthmatics[3]	% male[3,4]	Age[3,5]	Includes smokers[3,6]
Mannino et al., 2002	Nationwide	USA	523	59	4-16	No
Chapman et al., 2003			(309)	(60)	(8-16)	Never[13]
Morkjaroenpong et al., 2002	Baltimore and Washington DC	USA	590	40	5-11	NK
Wamboldt et al., 2002	Denver	USA	152	57	7-18	No[14]
Karadag et al., 2003	Istanbul	Turkey	32	63	1-14	NK
Soussan et al., 2003	Nationwide	France	167	64	6-12	NK
Halterman et al., 2004	Rochester, NY	USA	184	63	3-7	NK

1 Publications marked with an asterisk are abstracts.
2 Where there are multiple publications from the same study, the publications are shown together in the table with the location and country shown only for the earliest.
3 Where there are multiple publications from the same study, the value shown not in brackets is that used for the distributions discussed in the text.
4 NK = not known.
5 Age range is shown if available, otherwise mean preceded by mn, or median preceded by md.
6 NK = not known, No = no current smokers, Never = no ever smokers, number = number of known smokers included in analysis.
7 In follow-up phase. Selected from 400 asthmatics.
8 141 with a maternal report of an asthmatic attack, 134 with a diagnosis of asthma or wheezy bronchitis.
9 96% were aged 10-11.
10 5% of all children, not of all asthmatic children, were smokers.
11 Approximate estimate.
12 48% were aged <1.
13 Never or <5 packs during life.
14 Children were asked if they smoked, but the number who did was not stated.

Smoking habits. For 33 of the 47 studies (70%) no mention was made of smoking by the child, though some were based on children so young that smoking could effectively be ruled out. For one study, attention was restricted to children reported never to have smoked (Venners et al., 2001) and one publication from NHANES III (Chapman et al., 2003) was restricted to children with a lifetime consumption of 5 packs at most. In another analysis from NHANES III (Mannino et al., 2002) and in nine other studies (indicated by "No" in the final column in Table 1) current smokers were excluded. In three studies, and in an early analysis from the Vancouver study (Murray and Morrison, 1986), a few smokers were included in the analysis. The largest proportion of smokers was the 5% of all subjects in the study reported by Hu et al. (1997), although the proportion of smokers among the asthmatics was unknown.

Study design and subject selection. Table 2 summarizes details of the study design and subject selection for the 47 studies of asthma exacerbation in children.

Table 2. Details of study design and subject selection for the exacerbation studies in children

Publication[1]	Study type	Identification of asthma cases
O'Connell and Logan, 1974	Cases followed for 6 mo to 2 yr	Random from clinic files, children affected by ETS followed
Aderele, 1982	Case	Consecutive cases at asthma clinic
Gortmaker et al., 1982	Population cross-sectional	Questionnaire (ever had asthma)
Fergusson and Horwood, 1985	Cohort – from birth to 6 yrs	Repeated questionnaire (physician diagnosis of asthma/wheezy bronchitis; maternal report of attack)
Murray and Morrison, 1986, Murray and Morrison, 1988, Murray and Morrison, 1989, Murray and Morrison, 1992, Murray and Morrison, 1993	Case	Consecutive referrals at allergy clinic
Evans et al., 1987	Case	From outpatient clinics
O'Connor et al., 1987	School cross-sectional, including all household members	Questionnaire (told by physician has asthma in last 12 months)
Martinez et al., 1988	School cross-sectional	Questionnaire (ever had asthma)
Weitzman et al., 1990b, Weitzman et al., 1990a	Population cross-sectional	Questionnaire (has asthma, had it for 3 months, not cured)
Lilienfeld et al., 1990, Ehrlich et al., 1992	Case-control	Acute: ER; non-acute: asthma clinic
Frischer et al., 1992, Frischer et al., 1993, Meinert et al., 1994	School cross-sectional	Questionnaire (physician-diagnosis of asthma or wheezy bronchitis)
Salmun et al., 1992, Chilmonczyk et al., 1993	Case	Routine visit to allergy asthma clinic
Ogborn et al., 1994	Within subject comparison during acute episode and when symptom-free 3-4 wks later	ER visit with acute asthma attack

Table 2. Details of study design and subject selection for the exacerbation studies in children (Continued)

Publication[1]	Study type	Identification of asthma cases
Abulhosn et al., 1995, Abulhosn et al., 1997	Cases followed for 1 mo	All admissions with asthma diagnosis only
Chan and Chen, 1995	Cases monitored for 6 mo	Not known
LeSon and Gershwin, 1995	Case	Asthma admission to tertiary-care medical centre
Strachan and Carey, 1995	Case-control (drawn from school cross-sectional, only cases relevant)	Questionnaire (12+ wheezing attacks, or an attack that limited speech, in last 12 months)
MacArthur et al., 1996	Cases followed for 12 mo	Two admissions to hospital within 12 mo (follow-up period starts at second admission)
Meijer et al., 1996	Experimental, of treatment withdrawal	Symptoms of asthma, increased total IgE and allergy to HDM but not others, FEV>70% and increased bronchial responsiveness. Recruited at school (no details)
Callén Blecua et al., 1997	Case	First visit to outpatient clinic
Hu et al., 1997	Population cross-sectional	Questionnaire (ever physician diagnosed asthma)
Seidler et al., 1998	Cases followed for 3 yr	Any contact with participating doctor in 6 month baseline phase and any contact with same doctor in 6 months follow-up phase
Dubus et al., 1998, Oddoze et al., 1999	Case	Referred to respiratory function laboratory
Shamssain and Shamsian, 1999	School cross-sectional	Questionnaire (ever had asthma)
Wafula et al., 1999	Case	Consecutive cases at clinic or ward with 2+ previous episodes of wheezing
Al-Ghamdy et al., 2000	Case	Consecutive cases at health care centres and clinics
El-Dahr et al., 2000	Intervention trial on cases of effect of cessation advice	Not known
Güler et al., 2000	Cases, followed for 1 yr	Not known
Gürkan et al., 2000	Cases (studied retrospectively for 13 mo – 4 yrs)	All first admissions for asthma during 3 yr period
Li et al., 2000	Population cross-sectional	Questionnaire (physician diagnosed asthma)

Table 2. Details of study design and subject selection for the exacerbation studies in children (Continued)

Publication[1]	Study type	Identification of asthma cases
Melén et al., 2000, Melén et al., 2001	Cases followed for 2 yrs	Referred to paediatric clinics
Ratageri et al., 2000	Case-control (only cases relevant)	Consecutive cases with severe or mild asthma at clinic of tertiary hospital
Schwartz et al., 2000	School cross-sectional (3 mo diary study)	Questionnaire (ever doctor-diagnosed asthma, or wheezing or shortness of breath with wheezing in last 12 mo)
Crombie et al., 2001	Case	From GP record (and previously took part in intervention trial of advice to reduce ETS)
Ehrlich et al., 2001	Case (drawn from school cross-sectional study)	Questionnaire (parent-reported asthma and 1+ symptom last 12 mo, or 4+ symptoms last 12 mo)
Mayo, 2001	Case	Admitted with acute exacerbation without infection
Venners et al., 2001	Case	Physician diagnosed (had to have at least one sibling and 0 or 1 parents with asthma)
Wilson et al., 2001b	Intervention trial on cases of advice to reduce ETS	Visited ER or urgent clinic or hospitalised for acute asthma in last yr, and ETS exposed
Dales et al., 2002	Cases (drawn from school cross-sectional study)	Questionnaire (ever physician-diagnosed asthma and symptoms, attack or medication in last 12 mo)
Gaspar et al., 2002	Case-control	All acute asthma ER admissions and matched outpatient cases
Kalaajieh, 2002	Cases followed for up to 8 yr	All acute ER admissions
Mannino et al., 2002, Chapman et al., 2003	Population cross-sectional	Questionnaire (ever physician diagnosed asthma)
Morkjaroenpong et al., 2002	Case	All children with asthma diagnosis on school health records
Wamboldt et al., 2002	Cases (drawn from cohort study)	From school (receiving daily medication) or from insurance records (medication in last 6 mo or visit to allergist in last yr) but excluding 6+ steroid bursts or 2+ hospitalisations in last yr, or ever intubated
Karadag et al., 2003	Comparison during acute episode and when symptom-free 4 wks later	Consecutive admissions to emergency clinic with acute asthma

Table 2. Details of study design and subject selection for the exacerbation studies in children (Continued)

Publication[1]	Study type	Identification of asthma cases
Soussan et al., 2003	Cases with 3 yr follow-up	First two cases of recently diagnosed asthma (excluding severe cases) at each chest specialist in France, and on anti-inflammatory medication at 12 mo follow-up
Halterman et al., 2004	Intervention trial on cases of school-based provision of medication	All children with 2+ symptom days/wk, 2+ symptom nights/mo, 3+ acute visits in last yr or 1+ hospitalisation in last yr identified from school medical records.

ER = Emergency room or department.

[1] Multiple publications from the same study are separated by commas.

The majority of the studies fall into two broad classes, studies of asthma *cases* identified through medical records, and *cross-sectional* studies of children generally with the classification of asthma being based on questionnaire. There are 24 studies in the first class, of which 9 included an element of follow-up. For some of these studies the cases had been identified from a previous cross-sectional study or cohort study, or were part of a case-control study. There are 13 studies in the second class, 8 involving surveys in schools (one with follow-up) and 5 surveys in the general population.

There are five rarer study designs:

- One *cohort* study (Fergusson and Horwood, 1985) which followed children from birth to 6 years with repeated questionnaires used to identify asthmatics;
- Three *case-control* studies (Ehrlich et al., 1992; Ratageri et al., 2000; Gaspar et al., 2002) which compared groups of cases with differing asthma presentation (acute vs non-acute or mild vs severe);
- Two *within-person* studies (Ogborn et al., 1994; Karadag et al., 2003) in which children were compared while having an acute attack and later, when symptom-free;
- Three *intervention* studies (El-Dahr et al., 2000; Wilson et al., 2001b; Halterman et al., 2004) which investigated effects of advice to reduce ETS exposure or of school-based provision of medication; and
- One *experimental* study (Meijer et al., 1996) which investigated effects of treatment withdrawal.

Apart from giving information on broad study design, Table 2 makes clear the wide variety of definitions of asthma used in the studies, whether based on questionnaire or on medical records.

Markers of exposure. Table 3 shows for each study whether data are available by ETS exposure, by a cotinine-based marker or by exposure during gestation, as well as giving details of the actual exposure indices used. Of the 47 studies, all but three (marked by a dash in the relevant column) reported results for an index of ETS exposure. Although a few of the studies presented results specifically relating to maternal smoking, most considered smoking by other household members, including the father. Relatively few considered exposure outside the home, such as at day care (Chilmonczyk et al., 1993) or in all locations (Ogborn et al., 1994). Rather more studies took into account not only whether household members smoke, but also whether the smoking occurred inside the home. Eight studies reported results for a cotinine based marker, in most cases based on urine samples, though one study reported results based on saliva cotinine (Crombie et al., 2001) and one on serum cotinine (Mannino et al., 2002).

Adjustment for potential confounding variables. Of the 47 studies, 23 (49%) did not adjust for any potential confounding variables at all, not even age.

One of these (Ogborn et al., 1994) was a study of changes within child, where adjustment was not relevant. There were also some studies where the groups being compared were noted to be similar in respect of certain variables – such as sex, age, ethnicity and SES (Ehrlich et al., 1992); sex, age and asthma severity (Abulhosn et al., 1997); or body mass index (Dubus et al., 1998) – but in most of these the issues of confounding by other variables had not been addressed at all.

Table 4 gives details of the potential confounding variables taken into account in the different studies. Where a variable is listed for a study, it was taken into account in some of the relevant analyses, though not necessarily in all. Variables indicated in parentheses were considered as potential confounders but found to make little difference, with the analyses presented not actually adjusting for them.

Of the 24 studies listed, two (Martinez et al., 1988; Frischer et al., 1992) involved children of such a limited age range that age adjustment was not needed, and one was a study of changes within child (Wilson et al., 2001b). Of the other 21, only five (Gortmaker et al., 1982; Evans et al., 1987; Ratageri et al., 2000; Gaspar et al., 2002; Halterman et al., 2004) apparently ignored age.

Of the 23 between-child comparison studies considered in Table 4, 14 considered the sex of the child, with 10 actually presenting results adjusted for it.

Table 3. Indices of smoke exposure for which results are reported for the exacerbation studies in children

Publication[1]	Index of ETS exposure	Cotinine	Exposure during gestation
O'Connell and Logan, 1974	Parents quit or continued	-	-
Aderele, 1982	Household members smoke regularly	-	-
Gortmaker et al., 1982	Mother smokes	-	-
Fergusson and Horwood, 1985	Parents smoke	-	-
Murray and Morrison, 1986, 1988, 1989, 1992, 1993	Parents smoke	-	-
Evans et al., 1987	Household members smoke	-	-
O'Connor et al., 1987	Parents smoke	-	-
Martinez et al., 1988	Parents smoke	-	-
Weitzman et al., 1990b, 1990a	-		Mother
Lilienfeld et al., 1990, Ehrlich et al., 1992	Household members smoke	Urine CCR	-
Frischer et al., 1992, 1993, Meinert et al., 1994	Mother, Father smokes[2]	-	-
Salmun et al., 1992, Chilmonczyk et al., 1993	Household or day care smoking	Urine CCR	-
Ogborn et al., 1994	ETS in any location in last 48 hours	Urine cotinine, CCR	-
Abulhosn et al., 1995, 1997	Parents smoke	-	-
Chan and Chen, 1995	-	Urine CCR	-
LeSon and Gershwin, 1995	Parents, family, room-mates smoke	-	-
Strachan and Carey, 1995	Parents smoke (at home)	-	Mother[3]
MacArthur et al., 1996	Household members smoke	-	-
Meijer et al., 1996	Parents smoke	-	-
Callén Blecua et al., 1997	Parents smoke	-	-
Hu et al., 1997	Mother smokes	-	Mother
Seidler et al., 1998	Parents smoke (at home)	-	-
Dubus et al., 1998, Oddoze et al., 1999	Parents smoke[4]	Urine cotinine, CCR[4]	-
Shamssain and Shamsian, 1999	Parents smoke	-	-
Wafula et al., 1999	Household ETS	-	-
Al-Ghamdy et al., 2000	Parents smoke	-	-
El-Dahr et al., 2000	Parents smoking normally then reducing	-	-
Güler et al., 2000	Parents smoke	-	Mother[5]
Gürkan et al., 2000	Mother smokes, Indoor smoking (at home)	-	-
Li et al., 2000	Mother smokes	-	Mother

Table 3. Indices of smoke exposure for which results are reported for the exacerbation studies in children (Continued)

Publication[1]	Index of ETS exposure	Cotinine	Exposure during gestation
Melén et al., 2000, 2001	Parents smoke	-	-
Ratageri et al., 2000	Family members smoke	-	-
Schwartz et al., 2000	Smokers at home	-	-
Crombie et al., 2001	Parents smoke	Saliva cotinine	-
Ehrlich et al., 2001	Parents smoke	-	Mother[6]
Mayo, 2001	Parents 1+ pack/day	-	-
Venners et al., 2001	Father smokes[7]	-	-
Wilson et al., 2001b	Intervention vs usual care	-	-
Dales et al., 2002	Regular ETS at home	-	-
Gaspar et al., 2002	Household smoking	-	-
Kalaajieh, 2002	-	-	Household[8]
Mannino et al., 2002, Chapman et al., 2003	Smokers at home	Serum cotinine[9]	-
Morkjaroenpong et al., 2002	Caregiver smokes at home[10]	-	-
Wamboldt et al., 2002	Household members smoke	-	-
Karadag et al., 2003	Household members smoke	Urine cotinine	-
Soussan et al., 2003	Household members smoke (at home)	-	-
Halterman et al., 2004	Smokers at home	-	-

1 Multiple publications from the same study are separated by commas.
2 Results for father smoking only reported in Frischer et al., 1993.
3 Around time of birth.
4 Parental smoking and urinary CCR results only reported in Oddoze et al., 1999.
5 Also passive smoking by mother in pregnancy.
6 Also results relating to mother ever smoked and parents smoked in child's first year.
7 Mothers all never smokers and ex-smoking fathers excluded.
8 At birth.
9 Household smoking results only used in Chapman et al., 2003; cotinine results only reported in Mannino et al., 2002.
10 Caregivers who smoke, but not at home, excluded.

Table 4. Potential confounding variables taken into account in the exacerbation studies in children

Publication	Age[1]	Sex[1]	Others[1,2]
Gortmaker et al., 1982	No	No	Sample (= urban/rural)
Murray and Morrison, 1986, 1988, 1989, 1992, 1993	Yes	Yes	Recent respiratory infection, recent medication, positive skin test, family history of asthma, hot air heating, wood stove, gas range, pets, duration of asthma, age of onset of asthma, number of siblings, atopic dermatitis
Evans et al., 1987	No	No	Days with asthma symptoms per month
O'Connor et al., 1987	(Yes)	(Yes)	History of cold in last two weeks, predicted FEV, (height, atopy)
Martinez et al., 1988	All 9	Yes	Atopy
Frischer et al., 1992, 1993, Meinert et al., 1994	All 7-8	Yes	Prematurity, pneumonia in first year, atopy, education
Chilmonczyk et al., 1993	Yes	Yes	Day-care attendance, mother's age and education
Meijer et al., 1996	Yes	No	Pets, HDM exposure, PC_{20}
Seidler et al., 1998	Yes	Yes	Parental education, frequency of asthmatic episodes, infection-associated asthma, asthma on exertion, neurodermitis, hospitalisation, speciality of treating physician, parental asthma, sensitivity to exhaust gases, region
Gürkan et al., 2000	Yes	(Yes)	(Allergic conjunctivitis, eczema, frequent URI, familial allergy, +ve SPT, IgE, urban residency, using inhaled steroids)
Li et al., 2000	Yes	No	Community, school grade, spirometer, pressure, technician, height, race
Melén et al., 2000, 2001	Yes	No	Heredity, cat, dog, window condensation, 3+ SPT (possibly cat allergen, IgE cat, but not clear if univariate or multivariate)
Ratageri et al., 2000	No	No	Age of onset, past history lung disease, family history asthma, allergy, breastfeeding, overcrowding, pets, cooking, worm infestation, eosinophil count, air pollution
Schwartz et al., 2000	Yes	Yes	Height, weight, atopy, father's education, medication, day of study, weekend, temperature, humidity

Table 4. Potential confounding variables taken into account in the exacerbation studies in children (Continued)

Publication	Age[1]	Sex[1]	Others[1,2]
Crombie et al., 2001	Yes	(Yes)	Severity of asthma perceived and based on treatment step, number of children in family (parental age)
Ehrlich et al., 2001	Yes	Yes	Height, atopy, baseline FEV_1, asthma group, symptom score, medical insurance (parental education, mother contributes to income, hay fever, eczema, familial asthma)
Venners et al., 2001	Yes	No	Height, weight, father's education
Wilson et al., 2001b	No[3]	No[3]	Baseline outcome
Gaspar et al., 2002	No	No	Prior asthma hospitalisation, atopy, maternal asthma, last year asthma admission, onset of symptoms before 12 mo, attendance at day care or kindergarten, family size
Kalaajieh, 2002	(Yes)	(Yes)	Respiratory infections (atopic dermatitis, allergic rhinitis, IgE, eosinophil)
Mannino et al., 2002, Chapman et al., 2003	Yes	Yes	Race/ethnicity, SES, family size, parental history asthma, sitting height, parental history allergy or asthma, height, body mass, skinfold thickness, gas stove, income, pets, physical activity
Morkjaroenpong et al., 2002	Yes	No	Caregiver education, asthma primary care, medication
Soussan et al., 2003	Yes	Yes	Father's occupation, atopy, sensitisation to mites, cats/dogs, pollen and mould, perennial asthma, perennial/seasonal allergic rhinitis, atopic dermatitis, asthma in father, mother and sibs, gas cooking, mould, cat, dog, carpet, mattress type, medication compliance.
Halterman et al., 2004	No	(Yes)	(Baseline severity, baseline medication, race, ethnicity, parental age, parental education, poverty)

[1] Variables which were considered, found not to have any material confounding effect, but not adjusted for in any analysis are indicated by parentheses.

[2] The list of other variables considered is that taken into account in at least some relevant analysis. Not all analyses necessarily considered all of them.

[3] Within-child study so not necessary to adjust.

There are a wide variety of other factors taken into account in at least one study. The broad types of variables considered most commonly, with the number of studies adjusting for them (or determining that they did not have a material confounding effect) are as follows: child's medical history (18), family medical history or parental age (12), socio-economic status (SES) or parental education (9), height, weight or BMI (6), pets (5), location (including urban/rural) (5), family composition (4), and child's education or day care (4).

Not included among the variables listed in Table 4 are indices of ETS exposure. A few studies presented analyses linking an endpoint of interest to one index of ETS exposure, while adjusting for another (O'Connor et al., 1987; Murray and Morrison, 1988; Murray and Morrison, 1989; Frischer et al., 1992; Crombie et al., 2001).

Chapter 2

2. Results

2.1. Asthma Exacerbation and Severity

A wide variety of indices of asthma exacerbation and severity have been used. These have been classified into nine groups, with results presented in Tables 5 to 13.

The layout of each table is similar, with columns for publication, endpoint, exposure and result. In the simplest case there is a single endpoint and single exposure with the result usually expressed as an OR comparing the exposed and unexposed or as means for the exposed and unexposed. In some cases the comparison is different, e.g. highest vs lowest cotinine group, but this is made clear in the tables. Where results are given by level of endpoint (e.g. mild, moderate, severe asthma) or by level of exposure (e.g. 0, 1-9, 10+ cigs/day by the mother) the results are presented relative to a defined comparison (base) group. Where 95% confidence intervals are not available, p values are presented as $p<0.001$, $p<0.01$, $p<0.05$ or NS ($p\geq0.05$).

Each table in general presents a single set of results per study. Where there are multiple publications from the same study, the results selected are generally those based on the largest number of subjects, with data given in papers preferred to data given in abstracts.

Hospitalisation: Table 5

Nine studies have related hospital admissions, or in one study (Dales et al., 2002) hospitalisations or emergency department visits, to ETS exposure. Four of these (Gürkan et al., 2000; Mayo, 2001; Kalaajieh, 2002; Dales et al., 2002) reported a significant increase in frequency or length of admissions in relation to parental smoking or other indices of ETS exposure at home. A non-significant positive association was also seen in another study (MacArthur et al., 1996). Of the remaining four studies, two (Evans et al., 1987; Halterman et al., 2004) reported no significant association, but in fact provided little useful information, and one (Wilson et al., 2001b) reported a non-significant reduction in hospitalisation in the intervention group, which did not actually show any clear reduction in ETS exposure relative to the usual care group.

Table 5. Summary of results for children relating hospitalisation to ETS exposure

Publication	Endpoint	Exposure	Result[1]
Evans et al., 1987	Hospitalisation for asthma in last year	Household member smokes	Not significant (data not shown)
MacArthur et al., 1996	Readmission for asthma within a year	Household member smokes	OR 1.44 (0.87-2.37)
Gürkan et al., 2000	Multiple admissions per year	Mother smokes	OR 3.25 (1.13-8.85)[2]
		Indoor smoking at home	OR 2.55 (1.12-5.82)[3]
Mayo, 2001	Duration of stay for asthma	Parent(s) smoke 1+ pack/day	Mean 4.35 vs 2.86 days ($p<0.05$)
Wilson et al., 2001b	Hospitalisation for asthma in year	Intervention effect	OR 0.34 (NS)[4]
Dales et al., 2002	Hospitalisation for asthma or ER visit in last year	Regular ETS at home	OR 1.55 (1.22-1.97)
Kalaajieh, 2002	Multiple admissions for asthma per year	Mother smokes (at birth)	OR 6.10 (2.98-12.55)[5]
		Indoor smoking (at birth)	OR 3.06 (1.81-5.18)
Mannino et al., 2002	Hospitalisation for asthma in last year	Highest vs lowest cotinine[6]	OR 0.2 (0.1-0.5)[7]
		Intermediate vs lowest cotinine	OR similar to that for highest vs lowest, but NS
Halterman et al., 2004	Hospitalisation for asthma in study year	Smokers in home	OR 0.63 (0.15-2.58)

1 Unadjusted for covariates except where stated.

2 Adjusted for age (for mother smokes result only).

3 Indoor smoking found to be non-significant in multiple logistic regression analysis with maternal smoking already included in the model.

4 Intervention vs control, with adjustment for baseline differences.

5 OR for maternal smoking noted to be significant ($p<0.001$) in multiple logistic regression analysis, with recurrent URI the only other factor included, but OR not given.

6 Serum cotinine groups are 0.050 to 0.115 ng/ml = low, 0.116 to 0.639 ng/ml = intermediate, and 0.640 to 20 ng/ml = high.

7 Adjusted for age, race/ethnicity, SES, family size and parental history of asthma.

The final study (Mannino et al., 2002) reported a significantly *reduced* risk of hospitalisation for asthma in children with the highest cotinine levels. The authors considered that this negative association might have been because parents altered their smoking habits as a result of the hospitalisation, but this seems somewhat speculative. Their study generally found a tendency for cotinine to be positively associated with other asthma severity outcomes, and other studies, such as Dales et al., 2002, reported a positive association between current ETS exposure and previous hospitalisation. The explanation for this aberrant result, which conflicts with the general tendency of a positive relationship is unclear. However, as it was quite highly significant (OR = 0.2, 95% CI 0.1-0.5) and based on a nationally representative US sample from NHANES III, it should not be lightly dismissed.

Only one study (Weitzman et al., 1990b) reported findings for maternal smoking in pregnancy. This found that the mean number of overnight hospitalisations (from any cause) was unrelated to the number of cigarettes smoked by the mother (1.1, 1.3 and 1.0 for 0, 1-9 and 10+ cigs/day).

Emergency Room Visits: Table 6

Six studies have considered emergency room visits, urgent consultations or other related endpoints. Four of these also reported results for hospitalisations (Table 5), and for one of them (Dales et al., 2002) the data, for hospitalisations or emergency department visits, are the same as presented there. Three of the studies (Evans et al., 1987; LeSon and Gershwin, 1995; Dales et al., 2002) reported a significant positive association with ETS exposure, the most striking of which was the hugely strong relationship with whether the admission requires intubation (LeSon and Gershwin, 1995). A further study (Wilson et al., 2001b) also reported a significant reduction in acute medical visits in the intervention group though, as noted above, it was not clear if that group had in fact reduced ETS exposure. Other studies (Hu et al., 1997; Halterman et al., 2004) reported no significant association. In total, however, the data provide evidence of an association of emergency room visits with ETS exposure.

Only one study (Hu et al., 1997) has reported results for maternal smoking in pregnancy, finding no association.

Table 6. Summary of results in children relating emergency room visits and urgent consultations to ETS exposure

Publication	Endpoint	Exposure	Result[1]
Evans et al., 1987	ER visits for asthma in last year	Household member smokes	Mean 3.46 vs 2.12 ($p<0.01$)[2]
LeSon and Gershwin, 1995	Asthma admission requires intubation	ETS from parents, family members or room mates	OR 22.4 (7.4-68.0)[3]
Hu et al., 1997	ER visit for asthma in last year	Mother smoked in last week	OR 0.86 (0.40-1.89)
Wilson et al., 2001b	More than one acute medical visit for asthma in last year	Intervention effect	OR 0.32 ($p<0.05$)[4]
Dales et al., 2002	Hospitalisation for asthma or ER visit in last year	Regular ETS at home	OR 1.55 (1.22-1.97)
Halterman et al., 2004	3+ acute visits for asthma in study year	Smokers in home	OR 1.23 (0.62-2.43)

ER = emergency room or department

1 Unadjusted for covariates except where stated.

2 Adjusted for days with asthma symptoms per month.

3 From the data presented we estimate OR 22.2 (4.8-102.9).

4 Intervention vs control, with adjustment for baseline difference.

Restricted activity: Table 7

Six studies have related indices of restricted activity to ETS exposure. No significant association was reported in four studies (Gortmaker et al., 1982; Wilson et al., 2001b; Mannino et al., 2002; Morkjaroenpong et al., 2002). However one study (Halterman et al., 2004) reported significantly more school absences where there were smokers in the home, and another (El-Dahr et al., 2000) reported that the child had significantly more days with restricted activity during the three month period where the parents were smoking normally than during the following three month period after encouragement to quit smoking. The design of the latter study, reported only as an abstract, does not include a valid control group. The data for restricted activity, taken as a whole, do not demonstrate the existence of an association with ETS exposure.

No data are available relating restricted activity to exposure during gestation.

Table 7. Summary of results for children relating restricted activity to ETS exposure

Publication	Endpoint	Exposure	Result[1]
Gortmaker et al., 1982	Functional impairment[2]	Mother smokes cigarettes	OR 1.43 (0.79-2.65)[3]
El-Dahr et al., 2000	% days with restricted activity	Parent smoking normally, then reducing	10% vs 5% (p<0.05)
Wilson et al., 2001b	% with activity limitation in 2 wks before interview	Intervention effect	OR 0.64 (NS)[4]
Mannino et al., 2002	6+ school absences in last year	Highest vs lowest cotinine[5]	OR 1.8 (0.9-3.6)
		Intermediate vs lowest cotinine	OR similar to that for highest vs lowest, and NS
Morkjaroen-pong et al., 2002	Limited physical activity because of asthma in past 6 months	ETS exposure from caregiver:	OR
		0 cigs/day (base)	1.00
		1-9 cigs/day	0.57 (0.35-0.93)
		10+ cigs/day	1.03 (0.60-1.77)
		Any	0.74 (0.50-1.10)
	School days missed because of asthma in past 6 months	ETS exposure from caregiver:	Mean
		0 cigs/day (base)	6.7
		1-9 cigs/day	6.2 (NS)
		10+ cigs/day	8.4 (NS)
		Any	7.2 (NS)
Halterman et al., 2004	School absences because of asthma during study year	Smokers in home	Mean 10.28 vs 5.92 (p<0.01)

1 Unadjusted for covariates except where stated.
2 Functional impairment = affects ability to attend school or do any of the things a child of that age usually does.
3 Adjusted for study sample (= urban/rural).
4 Intervention vs control, with adjustment for baseline difference.
5 Serum cotinine groups are 0.050 to 0.115 ng/ml = low, 0.116 to 0.639 ng/ml = intermediate, and 0.640 to 20 ng/ml = high.

Acute and Non-Acute Asthma: Table 8

Two studies (Ogborn et al., 1994; Karadag et al., 2003) have compared ETS exposure in children at a time when they had an acute asthma attack and a few weeks later when they were well. Neither of these studies reported any significant increase in cotinine during the acute period, though one study (Ogborn et al., 1994) reported significantly increased reported ETS exposure based on one index, but not others. There were also two studies of case-control design (Ehrlich et al., 1992; Gaspar et al., 2002), where the cases were acute asthmatics and the controls non-acute asthmatics. The first of these reported no evidence of an association, but the second reported significant associations with various indices of ETS exposure, the strongest being the OR of 6.63 (2.5-17.8) for any ETS exposure. The overall data do not show a clear difference in ETS exposure between acutely and non-acutely asthmatic children.

No data were available relating acute and non-acute asthma to exposure during gestation.

Table 8. Summary of results comparing ETS exposure in acute and non-acute asthmatic children

Publication	Endpoint	Exposure	Result[1]
Ehrlich et al., 1992	Acute vs non-acute asthma (case-control study)	Any smoker in home	OR 0.84 (0.37-1.89)
		Cigs/day by all smokers	Mean 7.7 vs 10.7 (NS)
		Maternal caregiver smokes	OR 0.64 (0.28-1.44)
		CCR 30+ ng/mg	OR 0.90 (0.39-2.06)
		CCR ng/ml	Mean 46.2 vs 38.5 (NS)
Ogborn et al., 1994	Acute vs when well 3-4 wks later (within child comparison)	Cotinine (ng/ml)	Mean 81 vs 77 (NS)
		CCR (ng/mg)	Mean 93 vs 97 (NS)
		CCR 30+ ng/mg	80% vs 82% (NS)
		Hours exposed in last 48 hrs	Mean 32 vs 32 (NS)
		N cigs smoked at home in last 48 hrs	Mean 31 vs 25 (NS)
		ETS some or a lot	56% vs 44% ($p<0.05$)
Gaspar et al., 2002	Acute vs outpatient asthmatics (case-control study)	Any ETS	OR 6.63 (2.5-17.8)[2]
		Parents smoke	OR 3.51 (2.1-6.0)
		Father smokes	OR 3.0 (1.8-4.9)
		Mother smokes	OR 1.8 (1.0-3.1)
		Other residents at home smoke	OR 1.28 (0.8-2.0)
Karadag et al., 2003	Acute vs when well 4 wks later (within child comparison)	Cotinine (ng/ml)	Mean 295 vs 229.6 (NS)
		CCR (ng/mg)	Mean 314.6 vs 203.8 (NS)
		CCR 30+ ng/mg	81% vs 96% (NS)

1 Unadjusted for covariates except where stated.

2 For exposure "Any ETS" only, the OR is adjusted for the variables given in Table 4.

Asthma Medication: Table 9

Seven studies have related use of asthma medication to ETS exposure. In one study of children hospitalised for asthma (Abulhosn et al., 1997), beta-agonist therapy increased slightly over the 4 weeks following discharge among those living in homes where at least one parent smoked, while among those living in non-smoking homes it substantially reduced. In another study (Schwartz et al., 2000) a within-child analysis estimated that the odds of bronchodilator use were increased 10 fold in association with ETS exposure on the previous day. However, this estimate had very wide confidence limits of 1.3-38.7 and was only marginally significant. Another study (Murray and Morrison, 1988) also reported a marginally significant positive association of recent bronchodilator use with the number of cigarettes smoked by the mother, but not with the number smoked by the father. The other four studies cited in Table 9 reported no significant association or indeed any consistent tendency for asthma medication to be increased where ETS exposure was present. The overall data in Table 9 do not clearly demonstrate an association of ETS exposure with use of asthma medication.

Table 9. Summary of results for children relating use of asthma medication to ETS exposure

Publication	Endpoint	Exposure	Result[1]
Murray and Morrison, 1988	Recent bronchodilator use	N cigs smoked by mother	Correlation r = 0.12 (p = 0.04)
		N cigs smoked by father	Correlation r = -0.05 (NS)
Abulhosn et al., 1997	Reduction in beta-agonist therapy following hospital discharge (treatments in week 1 and week 4)	Smoking by parents	From 15.3 to 18.0 vs 20.8 to 8.9 (p<0.001)
Hu et al., 1997	Medication in last 2 wks	Mother smoked in last week	OR 0.67 (0.30-1.52)
Dubus et al., 1998	Anti-inflammatory treatment	Detectable cotinine	OR 0.66 (0.19-2.35)
El-Dahr et al., 2000	Bronchodilator use	Parent smoking normally, then reducing	Use said to decrease, but data inconsistent and no statement of significance
Schwartz et al., 2000	Bronchodilator use	ETS on previous day	OR = 10.3 (1.3-38.7)[2]
Halterman et al., 2004	Days using rescue inhaler per 14 days	Smokers in home	Mean 2.51 vs 1.97 (NS)

[1] Unadjusted for covariates except where stated.

[2] Adjusted for child (within-child analysis).

In one of the studies considered in Table 9 (Hu et al., 1997) use of medication was found not to be associated with maternal smoking in pregnancy. Another study (Weitzman et al., 1990b) reported some positive association between current use of asthma medication and maternal smoking in pregnancy. This was not significant for overall smoking, OR 1.75 (0.75-4.07), but was significant for smoking of 10+ cigs/day by the mother, OR 2.66 (1.02-6.91).

Health Contacts for Asthma: Table 10

Three studies have related ETS exposure to frequency of health contacts. Two studies have reported a somewhat higher frequency of contacts in the most ETS exposed children. In one of these (Fergusson and Horwood, 1985) the increase in frequency was only moderate, and the statistical significance was not known, and in the other (Mannino et al., 2002) the excess was larger but not statistically significant. In the third study (Crombie et al., 2001), no significant relationship was seen with cotinine level, but a statistically significant *negative* relationship was seen with three questionnaire-based indices of ETS exposure. The authors of this study, which was restricted to children with at least one smoking parent, suggested that *"this could be due to a lack of awareness of asthma symptoms among heavy smokers or a reluctance to visit the GP."* Factors such as social class or education, which one might expect to be correlated with awareness of asthma symptoms or reluctance to visit the GP, were not adjusted for in this study. It is strange that the multivariate analysis included both cotinine and parental smoking, two correlated markers of ETS exposure. The interpretation of such an analysis is not straightforward. Clearly the overall data do not demonstrate an increase in health contacts in relation to ETS exposure.

No information is available relating health contacts to exposure during gestation.

Asthma Severity: Table 11

Twelve studies have related ETS exposure to severity of asthma. In one early study (O'Connell and Logan, 1974) significantly increased asthma improvement was seen in children of parents who quit smoking compared to children whose parents continued to smoke. The other 11 studies have related asthma severity to indices of current ETS exposure. Significant positive associations were reported in seven of these studies (Aderele, 1982; Murray and Morrison, 1993; Strachan and Carey, 1995; Callén Blecua et al., 1997; Güler et al., 2000; Al-Ghamdy et al., 2000; Mannino et al., 2002), with non-significant positive associations seen in the remaining four, generally smaller, studies (Wafula et al., 1999; Ratageri et al., 2000; Melén et al., 2001; Wamboldt et al., 2002). However, in those studies that did report significant associations, the associations were not always significant (or even positive) in all analyses. This is most notably evident in the Vancouver study (Murray and Morrison, 1993), where a highly significant ($p<0.001$) positive association between asthma severity and maternal smoking was seen in children studied before July 1986, but a significant ($p<0.05$) *negative* association was seen in children studied later. Also in another study (Aderele, 1982) a significant positive association was seen if the father or older sibling smoked while a non-significant negative association was seen if other household members smoked. Overall, however, the data clearly show a positive association.

Only one study (Güler et al., 2000) related asthma severity to exposure during gestation, finding a significant ($p<0.01$) relationship with the number of cigarettes smoked by the mother.

Asthma Symptoms and Acute Episodes: Table 12

Fourteen studies have related asthma symptoms or acute attacks to ETS exposure. In six of the studies (Evans et al., 1987; Dubus et al., 1998; Shamssain and Shamsian, 1999; Ehrlich et al., 2001; Wilson et al., 2001b; Morkjaroenpong et al., 2002) no significant effect was seen and in another (Fergusson and Horwood, 1985) the pattern of results did not seem consistent with an association, though significance could not be estimated. In another study (Seidler et al., 1998) an increase in frequency of attacks associated with smoking by the parents was only marginally significant ($p=0.05$). The other six studies have reported a significant association for at least some of the relevant endpoints studied. By far the strongest associations seen were the about 10 fold increase in cough and phlegm related to smoking in the home in the last two days in the daily diary study in Finland (Schwartz et al., 2000). Significant associations with ETS exposure were also noted with frequency of acute exacerbations (Chilmonczyk et al., 1993), frequency of symptomatic days, but not symptomatic nights (Abulhosn et al., 1997), days with disturbed sleep and with cough, but not wheeze (El-Dahr et al., 2000), lack of symptom control (Soussan et al., 2003) and frequency of symptomatic days and nights (Halterman et al., 2004). Of the three studies that studied cotinine as a marker, one reported an association, with acute exacerbations

(Chilmonczyk et al., 1993) and two did not, with crises (Dubus et al., 1998) and with a symptom score (Ehrlich et al., 2001). While the overall results are certainly heterogeneous they are clearly strongly suggestive of an association.

None of the studies relate asthma symptoms and acute episodes to exposure during gestation.

Quality of Life and General Health: Table 13

Two studies have related ETS exposure to AQOL. In one study (Wamboldt et al., 2002) children with a smoker in the household had a non-significantly lower AQOL as assessed by the child but a significantly lower AQOL as assessed by the parent. In the other study (Halterman et al., 2004) no association was seen between ETS exposure and change in AQOL (in the intervention and usual care groups combined). Table 13 also includes results from one study (Mannino et al., 2002) showing no significant relationship of cotinine level to general health. This endpoint is clearly not very directly related to asthma specifically. These data are too limited for any useful conclusions to be drawn.

Summary of Results Presented in Tables 5 to 13

The data presented in Tables 5 to 13 relate to a wide variety of endpoints and indices of exposure, with results presented in various ways. Formal meta-analysis of the combined data is not practical. However Table 14 summarizes the results for each study in Tables 5 to 13 on a symmetrical 7 point scale as follows:

1. Decrease in risk – significant at $p<0.05$
2. Decrease in risk – not significant – by more than a factor of 1.5
3. Decrease in risk – not significant – by at most a factor of 1.5
4. No effect (association stated to be not significant but data not shown)
5. Increase in risk – not significant – by at most a factor of 1.5
6. Increase in risk – not significant – by more than a factor of 1.5
7. Increase in risk – significant at $p<0.05$

Table 10. Summary of results for children relating health contacts for asthma to ETS exposure

Publication	Endpoint	Exposure	Result[1]
Fergusson and Horwood, 1985	Annual rate of medical consultations for asthma per asthmatic child	Mother smokes cigarettes:	Rate
		None	0.80
		1-10/day	0.53
		11+/day	0.96 (Sig NK)
		Father smokes cigarettes:	Rate
		None	0.82
		1-10/day	0.64
		11+/day	0.85 (Sig NK)
Crombie et al., 2001	Health contacts for asthma (GP, medication, asthma clinic) in last 12 mo	No. of parents who smoke:	IRR[2]
		Father only (base)	1.00
		Mother only	0.76 (0.64-0.89)
		Both parents	0.78 (0.66-0.93)
		Child cotinine level:	IRR
		≤2.0 ng/ml (base)	1.00
		2.1-4.5 ng/ml	0.95 (0.82-1.11)
		>4.5 ng/ml	1.15 (0.98-1.34)
		Amount smoked in home by index parent:	IRR
		0-5 cigs/day (base)	1.00
		6-10 cigs/day	0.81 (0.71-0.92)
		11-15 cigs/day	0.70 (0.59-0.83)
		16-20 cigs/day	0.74 (0.61-0.91)
		>20 cigs/day	0.66 (0.47-0.93)
		Frequency of smoking in room with child:	IRR
		Never (base)	1.00
		Occasionally	0.76 (0.64-0.91)
		Frequently	0.60 (0.48-0.75)
		Every day	0.66 (0.56-0.77)
Mannino et al., 2002	Physician visit in last year for asthma	Highest vs lowest cotinine[3]	OR 1.80 (0.9-3.8)[4]
		Intermediate vs lowest cotinine	OR similar to that for highest vs lowest, and NS

1 Unadjusted for covariates except where stated.

2 IRR = incidence rate ratio. Results for number of parents who smoke and child cotinine level are from multivariate analysis which also includes age of child, perceived severity of asthma, severity of asthma by British Thoracic Society (BTS) treatment step and number of children in family. The study was restricted to children where at least one parent smoked.

3 Serum cotinine groups are 0.050 to 0.115 ng/ml = low, 0.116 to 0.639 ng/ml = intermediate, and 0.640 to 20 ng/ml = high.

4 Adjusted for age, race/ethnicity, SES, family size and parental history of asthma.

Table 11. Summary of results for children relating asthma severity to ETS exposure

Publication	Endpoint	Exposure	Result[1]
O'Connell and Logan, 1974	Asthma improved (basis not known)	Parent quit smoking	RR 3.38 (1.44-7.91)
Aderele, 1982	Severity of asthma (basis not known):	Household adult smokes regularly	OR
	Mild (base)		1.00 (base)
	Moderate		1.20 (0.67-2.15)
	Severe		1.48 (0.87-2.53)
		Father or older sib smokes regularly	OR
	Mild (base)		1.00 (base)
	Moderate		1.79 (0.87-3.67)
	Severe		2.61 (1.37-4.96)
		Other smoker in household	OR
	Mild (base)		1.00 (base)
	Moderate		0.68 (0.28-1.67)
	Severe		0.50 (0.20-1.29)
Murray and Morrison, 1993	Severity score (based on wheeze, wheeze on exertion, medication)	*Whole study period*	
		Cigs/day by mother	Correlation +0.19 (p<0.05)
		Cigs/day by father (in same room)	Correlation –0.04 (NS)
		Before July 1986	
		Mother smokes	Mean 8.2 vs 6.4 (p<0.001)
		Father smokes	Mean 7.1 vs 6.7 (NS)
		After July 1986	
		Mother smokes	Mean 5.8 vs 6.6 (p<0.05)
		Father smokes	Mean 6.5 vs 6.3 (NS)
Strachan and Carey, 1995	Frequent and speech-limiting attacks vs only one of these	Mother smokes now[2]:	OR
		0 cigs/day (base)	1.00
		1-10 cigs/day	1.69 (0.99-2.88)
		>10 cigs/day	1.86 (0.91-3.77)
		Any	1.74 (1.10-2.76)
		Father smokes now:	OR
		0 cigs/day (base)	1.00
		1-10 cigs/day	1.70 (0.93-3.12)
		>10 cigs/day	1.66 (0.73-3.77)
		Any	1.69 (1.01-2.82)
Callén Blecua et al., 1997	Severe (based on FVC, FEV_1, PEFR and $FEF_{25-75\%}$)	Parents smoke	OR 1.84 (1.12-3.03)

Table 11. Summary of results for children relating asthma severity to ETS exposure (Continued)

Publication	Endpoint	Exposure	Result[1]
Wafula et al., 1999	Severity (based on frequency of attacks):	Any smoking at home	OR
	Mild (base)		1.00
	Moderate		2.06 (0.96-4.40)
	Severe		Not given
Al-Ghamdy et al., 2000	Severity (based on Saudi national protocol):	Parents smoke	OR
	Mild (base)		1.00
	Moderate		1.81 (1.08-3.03)
	Severe		2.08 (1.25-3.46)
Güler et al., 2000	Severity score (basis unknown)	N cigs smoked by mother	Correlation p<0.01
		N cigs smoked by father	Correlation p<0.05
		CCR	NS (data not shown)
Ratageri et al., 2000	Severe (= wheeze most days/nights, restricted activity, growth affected, frequent medication) vs mild	Any family member smokes:	OR[3]
		0 cigs/day (base)	1.00
		1-9 cigs/day	0.66 (0.23-1.90)
		10+ cigs/day	2.22 (0.98-5.01)
		Any	1.49 (0.73-3.07)
		Father smokes	1.62 (0.78-3.35)
		Grandfather smokes	1.22 (0.35-4.24)
Melén et al., 2001	Severe (based on inhibited daily activity and steroid use in last year) vs mild/moderate	Smoking at home	OR 3.01 (0.74-12.2)[4]
Mannino et al., 2002	Severity (based on frequency of symptoms/respiratory illnesses in last year):		OR
	Moderate/severe vs mild	Highest vs lowest cotinine[5]	2.7 (1.1-6.8)
	Severe vs moderate/mild		1.9 (0.6-5.7)
		Intermediate vs lowest cotinine	ORs similar to those for highest vs lowest, but NS
Wamboldt et al., 2002	Functional severity score	Smoker in household	Mean 8.00 vs 7.40 (NS)

1 Unadjusted for covariates except where stated.
2 Results stated to be similar for mother smoked at time of child's birth.
3 Unadjusted ORs. OR adjusted for the variables listed in Table 4 were not given, but were not significant.
4 Adjusted for age, heredity, cat, dog, and window condensation.
5 Serum cotinine groups are 0.050 to 0.115 ng/ml = low, 0.116 to 0.639 ng/ml = intermediate, and 0.640 to 20 ng/ml high.

Table 12. Summary of results for children relating asthma symptoms and acute episodes to ETS exposure

Publication	Endpoint	Exposure	Result[1]
Fergusson and Horwood, 1985	Asthmatic attacks (maternal report)	Mother smokes:	Annual rate (per asthmatic)
		0 cigs/day	1.59
		1-10 cigs/day	0.96
		11+ cigs/day	2.03 (Sig NK)
		Father smokes:	
		0 cigs/day	1.55
		1-10 cigs/day	1.60
		11+ cigs/day	1.46 (Sig NK)
Evans et al., 1987	Frequency of days with symptoms	Household member smokes	No significant effect
Chilmonczyk et al., 1993	Acute exacerbations in past 12 months	ETS exposure from household members or at day-care:	Mean
		None	2.2
		Mother or other	2.5
		Mother and other	3.9
		Change per category	+0.83 (+0.39 to +1.26)[2]
		CCR:	
		<10 ng/ml	2.1
		10-39 ng/ml	2.8
		>39 ng/ml	3.6
		Change per category	+0.63 (+0.10 to + 1.07)[2]
Abulhosn et al., 1997	Symptomatic days (in month following discharge)	Smoking by parents	Mean 3.3 vs 1.4 (p<0.05)
	2+ symptomatic days		RR 4.00 (1.08-14.75)
	Symptomatic nights		Mean 2.3 vs 1.4 (NS)
Seidler et al., 1998	Increase in frequency of asthma attacks during follow-up	Smoking by parents	OR 1.7 (1.0-3.0)[2]
Dubus et al., 1998	Crises per year	Detectable cotinine	Mean 4.1 vs 4.4 (NS)
	Symptoms between crises		OR 0.49 (0.15-1.60)
Shamssain and Shamsian, 1999	Speech limitation during wheezing attack in past 12 months	Parents smoking:	
		Neither	13.1%
		One parent	14.0%
		Both parents	15.0% (NS)
El-Dahr et al., 2000	Symptom score	Parents smoking normally, then reducing	Mean 1.00 vs 0.54 (p<0.05)
	Days with disturbed sleep		15% vs 9% (p<0.01)
	Days with cough		30% vs 13% (p<0.01)
	Days with wheeze		22% vs 15% (NS)

Table 12. Summary of results for children relating asthma symptoms and acute episodes to ETS exposure (Continued)

Publication	Endpoint	Exposure		Result[1]
Schwartz et al., 2000	Cough	Smoking in the home in last 2 days		OR 12.4 (2.4-63.3)
	Phlegm production			OR 7.8 (1.4-41.7)
Ehrlich et al., 2001	Symptom score 8-10 vs 4-7	CCR (ng/mg)		GMean 64.1 vs 72.8 (NS)
Wilson et al., 2001b	Symptom-free days per 2 wk	Intervention effect		Mean diff -0.22 (NS)[3]
	Nights awakened per 2 wk			Mean diff -0.37 (NS)[3]
Morkjaroenpong et al., 2002	Nocturnal symptoms at least 2 nights per month	ETS exposure from caregiver:		OR[4]
		0	cigs/day (base)	1.00
		1-9	cigs/day	0.51 (0.30-0.85)
		10+	cigs/day	1.31 (0.68-2.50)
		Any		0.75 (0.49-1.15)
Soussan et al., 2003	Symptom control[5]	Smoker in home		OR 0.34 (0.13-0.91)[6]
		Mother smokes in home		OR 0.53 (0.20-1.37)
Halterman et al., 2004	Symptom-free days per 2 wk	Smokers in home		Mean 9.69 vs 10.97 ($p<0.01$)
	Symptom days per 2 wk			Mean 3.07 vs 2.07 ($p<0.01$)
	Symptom nights per 2 wk			Mean 3.05 vs 2.05 ($p<0.01$)

1 Unadjusted for covariates except where stated.

2 Adjusted for the variables given in Table 4.

3 Intervention vs control, with adjustment for baseline differences.

4 ORs are unadjusted. The authors also report an OR, adjusted for the variables given in Table 4, of 2.83 (1.22-6.55) for 10+ vs 1-9 cigs/day. This illogical analysis has not been included in the main body of the table.

5 Symptom control is defined as diurnal and nocturnal asthma <1/wk and no symptoms between attacks at all visits in 2nd and 3rd years of follow up.

6 OR for smoker in the home is adjusted for the variables given in Table 4, but OR for mother smokes in the home is unadjusted.

Table 13. Summary of results for children relating quality of life and general health to ETS exposure

Publication	Endpoint	Exposure	Result[1]
Mannino et al., 2002	Less than very good health	Highest vs lowest cotinine[2]	OR 1.3 (0.7-2.5)
		Intermediate vs lowest cotinine	OR similar to that for highest vs lowest, and NS
Wamboldt et al., 2002	Parent-assessed AQOL[3]	Smoker in household	Mean 5.38 vs 6.13 (p<0.01)
	Child-assessed AQOL		Mean 5.61 vs 5.77 (NS)
Halterman et al., 2004	Change in AQOL[3] during study year	Smokers in home	Mean 0.55 vs 0.36 (NS)

[1] Unadjusted for covariates except where stated.

[2] Serum cotinine groups are 0.050 to 0.115 ng/ml = low, 0.116 to 0.639 ng/ml = intermediate, and 0.640 to 20 ng/ml = high.

[3] AQOL = Asthma-related qualify of life. Lower scores indicate poorer quality.

Table 14. Summary of associations presented in Tables 5 to 13

			Decreased risk			No effect	Increased risk		
				Not significant			Not significant		
Table	Endpoint	No of studies	Significant at p<0.05	by >1.5	by ≤1.5		by ≤1.5	by >1.5	Significant at p<0.05
5	Hospitalisation	9	1	1	0	1	1	1	4
6	ER visits and urgent consultations	6	0	0	1	0	1	0	4
7	Restricted activity	6	0	0	1[1]	0	1	2	2
8	Acute and non-acute asthma	4	0	0	0	0	3	0	1
9	Asthma medication	7	0	1	1	0	2[2]	0	3
10	Health contacts for asthma	3	0	0	0	0	2[3]	1	0
11	Asthma severity	13[4]	1	0	1	0	3	2	6[5]
12	Asthma symptoms and acute episodes	14	0	0	4[6]	1	1	1[3]	7[7]

13	AQOL and general health	3	0	0	1	0	1	0	1[8]
	TOTAL	64[9]	2	2	9	2	15	7	27[9]

ER = emergency room or department, AQOL = asthma-related quality of life

[1] Choosing data for limited physical activity from Morkjaroenpong et al. (2002).

[2] Including result for El-Dahr et al. (2000).

[3] Including results from Fergusson and Horwood (1985).

[4] Counting as two separate studies results before and after July 1986 from Murray and Morrison (1993).

[5] Including result for moderate/severe vs mild from Mannino et al. (2002).

[6] Choosing data for crises per year from Dubus et al. (1998) and from Wilson et al. (2001b).

[7] Choosing data for symptomatic days from Abulhosn et al. (1997) and for symptom score from El-Dahr et al. (2000).

[8] Choosing data for parent-assessed AQOL for Wamboldt et al. (2002).

[9] Only counting once the significant increase reported for Dales et al., 2002 in Tables 5 and 6

Here an "increase" not only includes cases where an increase in an adverse health effect (or a decrease in a beneficial health effect) was associated with ETS exposure, but where a reduction in risk of an adverse health effect was associated with intervention to reduce ETS exposure (El-Dahr et al., 2000; Wilson et al., 2001b). For each study in each table, only one result is counted. Where there is a choice of ETS exposure indices preference is given to those based on mean cotinine, mean CCR, total ETS exposure and smoking by the mother in that order. Results are normally included in Table 14 based on the exposed/unexposed result, but the highest exposure level is used if only dose-response data are available.

It is evident that the overall data in Table 14 are consistent with a positive association. Of the 64 results summarised, 27 show a significant positive association and only two (Murray and Morrison, 1993 for asthma severity for results after July 1986 and Mannino et al., 2002 for hospitalisation) a significant negative one. Similarly, there are seven non-significant increases by a factor of 1.5 or more as compared to two non-significant decreases by the same factor. While the data are heterogeneous, with many studies showing little effect if any and a few very strong relationships, it is clear the overall pattern of results is not due to chance. This conclusion would have been unaffected by alternative plausible rules for preferring which results to include from studies providing a choice of ETS exposure variables.

2.2. Lung Function

Table 15 summarizes results from 18 studies relating ETS exposure to five lung function variables: FEV_1, FVC, the ratio of FEV_1 to FVC, $FEF_{25\text{-}75\%}$ and PEFR.

FEV_1

Seven of the 12 studies providing data for FEV_1 reported no significant association with ETS exposure (Evans et al., 1987; O'Connor et al., 1987; Chilmonczyk et al., 1993; Callén Blecua et al., 1997; Dubus et al., 1998; Venners et al., 2001; Wilson et al., 2001b). In the Vancouver study (Murray and Morrison, 1993) no significant association of FEV_1 with parental smoking was seen for children studied after July 1986. However, for children born before July 1986, FEV_1 was significantly reduced if either the mother or the father smoked. In the Southern California study (Li et al., 2000), current smoking was not associated with FEV_1 but past ETS exposure was associated with a significantly ($p<0.05$) reduced FEV_1 in boys but not girls. In the Cape Town study (Ehrlich et al., 2001), current smoking by the mother was associated with a significantly ($p<0.05$) reduced FEV_1, but no significant association was seen with other indices of parental smoking or with cotinine. In the analyses based on NHANES III, no significant association was seen between FEV_1 and smoking at the home (Chapman et al., 2003) but FEV_1 was significantly lower in those with high cotinine (0.640+ ng/ml) than in those with low cotinine (<0.116 ng/ml) (Mannino et al., 2002). The most significant association seen ($p<0.001$) was in the New Orleans study (El-Dahr et al., 2000) where FEV_1 was found to improve in 15 out of 17 children when the parents reduced the amount they smoked. As noted previously, this study lacked a proper control group. Overall these data do not provide very clear evidence that ETS exposure is associated with reduced FEV_1.

FVC

Four of the studies with relevant data reported no significant association of FVC with ETS exposure (O'Connor et al., 1987; Callén Blecua et al., 1997; Dubus et al., 1998; Venners et al., 2001). In the Vancouver study (Murray and Morrison, 1989) no relationship was seen with maternal smoking, but a marginally significant ($p=0.05$) reduced FVC was seen where the father smoked. In the study in Southern California (Li et al., 2000) no association of FVC with ETS exposure was seen in boys, but in girls, children with 2 or more current smokers in the household had a significantly ($p<0.05$) *increased* FVC. As for FEV_1, the results from NHANES III showed no association of FVC with the number of smokers in the home (Chapman et al., 2003) but did show a significantly ($p<0.05$) reduced FVC in the high cotinine group (Mannino et al., 2002). The combined data for FVC do not clearly demonstrate the existence of an association.

FEV_1/FVC

No significant association was reported in most studies (Callén Blecua et al., 1997; Venners et al., 2001; Mannino et al., 2002; Chapman et al., 2003). In the Southern California study (Li et al., 2000) a significantly ($p<0.05$) reduced FEV_1/FVC was seen in relation to past ETS exposure in boys, but no association was seen in relation to current smoking or in girls. The study in Portland (Chilmonczyk et al., 1993) reported a significant ($p<0.05$) reduction in FEV_1/FVC associated with household or day care smoking and cotinine. More data are needed to reach any clear conclusion here.

$FEF_{25-75\%}$

Of the eight studies providing evidence, three (Evans et al., 1987; O'Connor et al., 1987; Dubus et al., 1998) did not find a significant association of $FEF_{25-75\%}$ with ETS exposure. The remaining five did report a significant association, but often only in some analyses. Thus the Vancouver study (Murray and Morrison, 1993) reported a highly significant ($p<0.001$) reduction if the mother smoked for children born before July 1986, but a non-significant increase for children born after July 1986, and no association with father smoking in either period. Also, while the study in Southern California (Li et al., 2000) reported a significant ($p<0.05$) reduction in boys but not girls (and then only in relation to past but not current ETS exposure), the NHANES III study (Chapman et al., 2003) reported a significant ($p<0.05$) reduction in girls but not boys associated with having two smokers in the home. Significant ($p<0.05$) reductions were also reported in NHANES III (Mannino et al., 2002) in relation to cotinine level, and in the Portland study (Chilmonczyk et al., 1993) in relation to household or day care smoking and cotinine. The significant results for $FEF_{25-75\%}$ from the Istanbul study (Güler et al., 2000) are for increased reversibility and are not directly comparable to the other data. Overall, the data for $FEF_{25-75\%}$ are more suggestive of an association with ETS than is the case for FEV_1, FVC or FEV_1, but there are still inconsistencies which need resolution.

PEFR

The data included in Table 15, from 10 studies, are for a variety of endpoints, including PEFR variability (Frischer et al., 1993), PEFR amplitude (Meijer et al., 1996), PEFR reversibility (Güler et al., 2000) and PEF control (Soussan et al.,

2003) as well as PEFR level (Evans et al., 1987; Chan and Chen, 1995; Callén Blecua et al., 1997; Dubus et al., 1998; Schwartz et al., 2000; El-Dahr et al., 2000). Of the five studies where significant associations were noted, three (Chan and Chen, 1995; El-Dahr et al., 2000; Güler et al., 2000) were only incompletely reported in abstracts, one (Frischer et al., 1993) reported an association only in non-atopic children and one (Chan and Chen, 1995) reported an association with cotinine only for samples collected at night and not during the day. The study in Finland (Schwartz et al., 2000) reported a significantly ($p<0.05$) reduced PEFR associated with ETS exposure in between-child comparisons, but not in within-child comparisons. Taken as a whole, these data are difficult to interpret.

Other Lung Function Variables

There are very limited data for other lung function variables that are not shown in Table 15. In the study in Marseilles (Dubus et al., 1998; Oddoze et al., 1999) no association was found between cotinine level and SRAW. In NHANES III (Chapman et al., 2003) $FEF_{25-75\%}$/FVC was not associated with smoking in the household in boys (levels 0.791, 0.771, 0.796 for 0, 1, 2+ smokers in the home) but was significantly ($p<0.05$) lower in more heavily exposed girls (levels 1.265, 1.243, 1.054).

Overall Conclusions for Lung Function

While there are a number of statistically significant findings in Table 15, the data generally do not show a very consistent pattern. Often associations are seen only for subsets of the data (Murray and Morrison, 1993; Chan and Chen, 1995; Meijer et al., 1996; Li et al., 2000; Chapman et al., 2003) or for some indices of exposure and not others (Murray and Morrison, 1993; Schwartz et al., 2000; Li et al., 2000; Ehrlich et al., 2001), with some studies reporting no significant associations at all (Evans et al., 1987; O'Connor et al., 1987; Callén Blecua et al., 1997; Dubus et al., 1998; Venners et al., 2001; Wilson et al., 2001b; Soussan et al., 2003). A clear relationship of ETS exposure to reduced lung function has not been established, though the data are somewhat suggestive of a relationship, particularly for $FEF_{25-75\%}$.

Table 15. Summary of results for children relating lung function to ETS exposure

Publication	Exposure	Lung function variable				
		FEV_1	FVC	FEV_1/FVC	$FEF_{25-75\%}$[1]	PEFR
Evans et al., 1987	No household smoker	1.49ℓ			1.42ℓ/sec	2.74ℓ/sec
	Household smoker	1.60ℓ			1.60ℓ/sec	3.19ℓ/sec
	p	NS			NS	NS
O'Connor et al., 1987	Mother non-smoker	102.9%	104.0%		85.8%	
	Mother smoker	100.8%	107.8%		76.1%	
	p	NS	NS		NS	
Frischer et al., 1993	Effects of mother smoking in non-atopic children					+54.7%[2], $p<0.05$
	Effect of mother smoking in atopic children					-8.5%[2], NS
Chilmonczyk et al., 1993	No household or day-care smoker	109.3%		83.7%	85.4%	
	Mother or others smoke	102.4%		79.4%	71.8%	
	Mother and others smoke	102.2%		80.0%	73.6%	
	Trend p	NS		$p<0.05$	$p<0.05$	
	Cotinine <10 ng/ml	108.8%		83.5%	85.4%	
	10-39 ng/ml	105.2%		81.2%	74.9%	
	40+ ng/ml	98.5%		77.5%	67.3%	
	Trend p	NS		$p<0.05$	$p<0.05$	
Murray and Morrison, 1993 (FVC data are from Murray and Morrison, 1989)	*Before July 1986:*					
	Mother non-smoker	84.4%	93.8%		71.7%	
	Mother smoker	77.3%	91.2%		59.5%	
	p	$p<0.01$	NS		$p<0.001$	
	Father non-smoker	84.2%	94.5%		70.0%	
	Father smoker	80.2%	90.6%		67.1%	
	p	$p<0.05$	$p=0.05$		NS	

Table 15. Summary of results for children relating lung function to ETS exposure (Continued)

Publication	Exposure	Lung function variable				
		FEV_1	FVC	FEV_1/FVC	$FEF_{25\text{-}75\%}$[1]	PEFR
Murray and Morrison, 1993 (continued)	*After July 1986:*					
	Mother non-smoker	90.8%			79.4%	
	Mother smoker	91.3%			81.0%	
	p	NS			NS	
	Father non-smoker	90.1%			78.0%	
	Father smoker	93.0%			84.1%	
	p	NS			NS	
Chan and Chen, 1995	Cotinine/creatinine ratio (CCR)					CCR significantly higher where PEFR<80% of predicted for samples collected at night, not during the day
Meijer et al., 1996	*During ICS*[3]*:*					
	Parents non-smokers					20.6%
	Parent smokes					28.7%
	p					NS
	After ICS withdrawal[3]*:*					
	Parents non-smokers					19.4%
	Parent smokes					29.7%
	p					$p<0.05$
Callén Blecua et al., 1997	Parents non-smokers	93.7%	97.4%	76.7%		92.6%
	Parent smokes	91.9%	96.9%	72.7%		87.2%
	p	NS	NS	NS		NS
Dubus et al., 1998	No cotinine	101.9%	101.7%		104.3%	85.6%
	Detectable cotinine	106.5%	106.6%		94.0%	89.1%
	p	NS	NS		NS	NS

Publication	Exposure	Lung function variable				
		FEV_1	FVC	FEV_1/FVC	$FEF_{25\text{-}75\%}$[1]	PEFR
El-Dahr et al., 2000	Parent smoking normally then reducing	Improved in 15/17				Improved in 8/15, worsened in 1/15
	p	<0.001				p<0.05
Güler et al., 2000[4]	Mother smokes now				Higher	?
	p				p=0.03	NS?
	Mother smoked in pregnancy				Higher	Higher
	p				p=0.001	Significant(NOS)
Li et al., 2000[5]	*Boys:* Past ETS	-4.9, p<0.05	-2.2, NS	-2.8, p<0.05	-9.2, p<0.05	
	One current smoker	-3.9, NS	-3.3, NS	-0.6, NS	-4.0, NS	
	Two+ current smokers	-2.9, NS	+0.8, NS	-3.6, NS	-5.2, NS	
	Girls: Past ETS	+2.1, NS	+2.5, NS	-0.2, NS	+1.4, NS	
	One current smoker	+1.1, NS	+1.9, NS	-0.8, NS	+7.0, NS	
	Two+ current smokers	+2.7, NS	+5.9, NS	-2.7, NS	-4.2, NS	
Schwartz et al., 2000[6]	Any ETS at home a.m.					-41.9 ℓ/min, p<0.05
	Any ETS at home p.m.					-40.7 ℓ/min, p<0.05
	ETS previous day					-9.2 ℓ/min, NS
Ehrlich et al., 2001	Mother not current smoker	1.64ℓ				
	Mother current smoker	1.41ℓ				
	p	p<0.05				
	Mother never smoked	1.47ℓ				
	Mother ever smoked	1.53ℓ				
	p	NS				
	Mother did not smoke in child's 1st yr	1.56ℓ				
	Mother smoked in child's 1st yr	1.46ℓ				
	p	NS				
	Father not current smoker	1.45ℓ				
	Father current smoker	1.56ℓ				

Table 15. Summary of results for children relating lung function to ETS exposure (Continued)

Publication	Exposure	Lung function variable: FEV_1	FVC	FEV_1/FVC	$FEF_{25-75\%}$[1]	PEFR
Ehrlich et al., 2001 (continued)	p	NS				
	Father did not smoke in child's 1st yr	1.50ℓ				
	Father smoked in child's 1st yr	1.52ℓ				
	p	NS				
	Not 2+ smokers in household	1.59ℓ				
	2+ smokers in household	1.46ℓ				
	p	NS				
	CCR 1st quartile	1.47ℓ				
	2nd quartile	1.47ℓ				
	3rd quartile	1.65ℓ				
	4th quartile	1.42ℓ				
	Trend p	NS				
Venners et al., 2001[7]	*Boys:* Father current <30 cigs/day	-1.9%, NS	-1.8%, NS	"No important association"		
	30+ cigs/day	-3.7%, NS	-3.7%, NS			
	Girls: Father current <30 cigs/day	-1.0%, NS	-0.4%, NS	"No important association"		
	30+ cigs/day	-1.3%, NS	-0.8%, NS			
Wilson et al., 2001b[8]	Intervention effect	-0.41%				
	p	NS				
Mannino et al., 2002[9]	Difference high vs low cotinine	-8.1%	-5.6%	-3.0%	-12.5%	
	p	p<0.05	p<0.05	NS	p<0.05	
	Difference intermediate vs low cotinine	Not given	Not given	Not given	Not given	

Publication	Exposure		Lung function variable				
			FEV_1	FVC	FEV_1/FVC	$FEF_{25-75\%}$[1]	PEFR
	p		NS	NS	NS	NS	
Chapman et al., 2003[10]	Boys: (base)	No smoking at home	2.61ℓ	3.16ℓ	82.6%	2.50 ℓ/s	
		1 smoker at home	2.65ℓ	3.21ℓ	82.5%	2.65 ℓ/s	
		p	NS	NS	NS	NS	
		2 smokers at home	2.39ℓ	2.93ℓ	81.5%	2.33 ℓ/s	
		p	NS	NS	NS	NS	
	Girls:	No smoking at home (base)	2.92ℓ	3.13ℓ	93.1%	3.96 ℓ/s	
		1 smoker at home	3.02ℓ	3.24ℓ	93.2%	4.03 ℓ/s	
		p	NS	NS	NS	NS	
		2 smokers at home	2.72ℓ	3.06ℓ	88.9%	3.22 ℓ/s	
		p	NS	NS	NS	$p<0.05$	
Soussan et al., 2003[11]	Smoker in home						OR 0.73 (0.39-1.38)
	Mother smokes at home						OR 0.34 (0.14-0.89)

1 Including MMEFR.
2 Data are percentage increase in PEFR variability in children with a smoking mother.
3 ICS = inhaled corticosteroids. PEFR values are PEFR amplitude = (maximum-minimum)/mean based on 24 hour data.
4 Data are for FEF and PEF reversibility. Significance not stated for PEF reversibility and smoking now but presumably not significant.
5 Data are percentage differences vs no ETS exposure and are irrespective of in utero exposure.
6 Data are average changes over a 3 month period. For any ETS exposure at home they derive from a between-child analysis, while for ETS previous day they derive from a within-child analysis.
7 Data are changes relative to father never smoker.
8 "Intervention effect" is change in intervention group from baseline to follow-up relative to corresponding change in usual care group.
9 Cotinine groups are 0.050 to 0.115 ng/ml = low, 0.116 to 0.639 ng/ml = intermediate, 0.640 to 20 ng/ml = high.
10 Values are model-predicted (see Chapman et al., 2003 Table 4).
11 Data are for PEF control (<20% variability) vs lack of control.

2.3. Bronchial Responsiveness

Seven studies have related ETS exposure to bronchial responsiveness.

In the Boston study (O'Connor et al., 1987) the response to cold air challenge (fall in FEV_1 as a percentage of predicted FEV_1) was greater if the mother smoked (24% vs 11.9% for mother non-smoker), but not if the father smoked (15% vs 17.1% for father non-smoker). The association with maternal smoking was significant ($p=0.02$) using one statistical technique, but not ($p=0.07$) using another.

In the Viterbo study (Martinez et al., 1988) the response to carbachol (fall of >20% FEV_1) was significantly ($p<0.05$) greater if the parents smoked, the OR being estimated as 18.7, but with a very wide confidence interval of 1.5 to 232.3.

In the Vancouver study bronchial responsiveness to histamine was reported to be significantly related to maternal but not paternal smoking in the first few papers describing results (Murray and Morrison, 1986; Murray and Morrison, 1988; Murray and Morrison, 1989; Murray and Morrison, 1992). In the final paper (Murray and Morrison, 1993) the increase in bronchial responsiveness (reduction in lung PC_{20}) in relation to maternal smoking was evident only in children examined before July 1986 (mother smoker –0.23, mother non-smoker +0.44, $p<0.05$) but not in children examined afterwards (+0.41 vs +0.26, NS). The same tendency was evident for father smoking (+0.12 vs +0.32, NS before July 1986; +0.74 vs +0.10, NS after July 1986).

In the Freiburg study (Frischer et al., 1992; Meinert et al., 1994) bronchial responsiveness to an exercise test (15% decrease in PEFR) was higher if the mother had smoked before pregnancy (OR 1.7) or had smoked when the child was 1 year old (OR 2.2), but was lower if the mother smoked when the test was done at age 8 (OR 0.5). These differences were non-significant in univariate analyses. Multivariate analyses implausibly claimed a significant 20 fold increase in bronchial responsiveness associated with maternal smoking at age 1 and a significant 20 fold decrease associated with maternal smoking at age 8. However these analyses are highly open to question because of the inter-correlations of the maternal smoking variables.

In the Marseilles study (Dubus et al., 1998) the response to carbachol (concentration to produce a 2-fold increase in SRAW) was significantly ($p<0.05$) decreased in children with a detectable cotinine (108.3 vs 160.9 for undetectable) but was non-significantly decreased if the mother smoked (98.4 vs 147.2 for father smoked or parents did not smoke). The percentage of bronchodilation was significantly ($p<0.05$) increased in children with a detectable cotinine (74.8 vs 68.8), but was not significantly related to parental smoking (data not given).

In the New Orleans study (El-Dahr et al., 2000) the response to methacholine challenge did not vary between the 3 month period where smokers in the child's household smoked normally and the 3 month period where they were encouraged to quit. 7 of 17 children improved, and 7 worsened, with the other 3 showing no change.

In the Cape Town study (Ehrlich et al., 2001) bronchial responsiveness to histamine (fall of >20% FEV_1) was found not to be significantly related to cotinine (OR 1.00, 0.86, 0.94, 0.81 for 4 quartiles) or a variety of indices of parental smoking (e.g. mother current smoker OR 0.78, CI 0.54-1.12 or father current smoker OR 0.99, CI 0.78-1.27).

Taken as a whole these data do not show a consistent relationship of ETS exposure to bronchial responsiveness.

Chapter 3

3. SUMMARY AND CONCLUSIONS

3.1. SUMMARY

Sixty relevant publications, apparently relating to 47 separate studies, were identified. 34 of the studies were first reported in the last 10 years (1995 to 2004). Results were available from a total of 22 countries, with more studies (18) conducted in the USA than in other countries. The median number of asthmatics studied was 167 per study, the largest study involving 3010. Studies generally were of both sexes, with more boys than girls. Most studies covered an age range of a few years, with 6-9 year olds most commonly studied. A few studies specifically excluded smokers.

There were a variety of study designs, including one experimental and three intervention studies, but most studies were of cases identified through medical records, or cross-sectional studies with the classification of asthma based on questionnaire. Eight of the 47 studies used a nicotine-based marker of ETS exposure, with other studies relying on questionnaire response. Only eight studies recorded maternal smoking in pregnancy.

About half the studies did not adjust for any potential confounding variables, with some potential confounding variables (such as diet, exercise and recent respiratory infections) rarely adjusted for.

A wide variety of indices of asthma exacerbation and severity were used in the studies, and the results are summarized under nine different endpoints. The endpoints, the number of studies providing data, the number showing a significant positive (negative) association with ETS exposure are summarized in the table on the next page.

Overall, these data show considerable evidence of an association, though the results appear heterogeneous, with a few studies reporting very strong relationships and a number no positive relationship at all. However, interpretation of this association is not straightforward for a number of reasons. These include the lack of clear evidence that increases in ETS exposure within child are associated with exacerbations of asthma, limited reporting of relevant study details by many authors (including information on active smoking by the child) and failure to separate out results by sex and by age. Failure to control for potential confounding variables is also a feature of the studies. No studies adjusted for maternal smoking in pregnancy, only six for any social class related variables, only four for infections in the child (and none for infections in the parent) and few even take the sex or age of the child into account. Furthermore, some of the various endpoints used may not be very direct or reliable measures of asthma severity.

Endpoint	Number of studies	Number significant +ve (-ve)	Conclusion/comment
Hospitalisation	9	4 (1)	Some evidence of an association, but data from NHANES III conflict
ER visits and urgent consultations	6	4 (0)	Evidence of an association
Restricted activity	6	2 (0)	Association not demonstrated
Acute and non-acute asthma	4	1 (0)	No clear difference in ETS exposure between acutely and non-acutely asthmatic children
Asthma medication	7	3 (0)	Association not clearly demonstrated.
Health contacts for asthma	3	0 (0)	No association shown
Asthma severity	13	6 (1)	Clear positive association
Asthma symptoms and acute episodes	14	7 (0)	Results heterogenous, but strongly suggestive of an association
AQOL and general health	3	1 (0)	Data too limited to draw conclusions
Total	64 [1]	27 [1] (2)	Overall data clearly show a positive association, not attributable to chance

ER = emergency room or department, AQOL = asthma-related quality of life.

[1] For one study, the same significant result has been reported under both the first two endpoints, but is only counted once in the totals.

Very few studies investigated these endpoints in relation to maternal smoking in pregnancy. There were five reported results, of which two (for asthma medication and severity) showed a significant positive association.

Eighteen studies related ETS exposure to one or more of five lung function variables – FEV_1, FVC, the ratio of FEV_1 to FVC, $FEF_{25\text{-}75\%}$ and PEFR. The data for $FEF_{25\text{-}75\%}$ are more suggestive of an association with ETS than is the case for FEV_1, FVC or the FEV_1/FVC ratio, but there are still inconsistencies which need resolution. The data on PEFR relate to a variety of endpoints, and the results, which are incompletely reported, are difficult to interpret. Other lung function variables have only very rarely been studied. While a number of statistically significant findings have been reported for lung function, the data generally do not show a very consistent pattern, with associations seen only for subsets of the data or for some indices of exposure and not others, with some studies reporting no significant associations at all. A clear relationship of ETS exposure to reduced lung function has not been established, though the data are somewhat suggestive of a relationship.

Seven studies have related ETS exposure to bronchial responsiveness, but no consistent association has been shown.

3.2. Other Reviews of the Evidence

An early review published by the Canadian Paediatric Society (Canadian Paediatric Society, 1986) was entitled *"Secondhand cigarette smoke worsens symptoms in children with asthma."* Although its conclusions were consistent with its title, only two of the 25 references cited actually concerned exacerbation of asthma. One was an experimental chamber study considered in Chapter 3 (Dahms et al., 1981), the other the study in Vancouver (Murray and Morrison, 1986) which reported that severity of asthma was increased if the mother smoked, but not if the father did. Most of the evidence cited related to healthy children, not asthmatics, so the conclusion that *"There is little doubt that cigarette smoke worsens asthma"* seems invalid, based on the evidence presented.

Ehrlich et al. (1993) published a review entitled *"Is passive smoking a cause of asthma in children?"* Although the authors noted the distinction between studies of asthma induction and studies of asthma exacerbation, the studies cited to support the conclusion that there is *"consistent evidence that among children already asthmatic, maternal smoking is associated with more severe asthma, more frequent visits to the emergency room, and greater bronchial hyperresponsiveness"* included a number not relevant to exacerbation. The only relevant studies cited were the series of studies in Vancouver (Murray and Morrison, 1986; Murray and Morrison, 1988; Murray and Morrison, 1989) and two others (Evans et al., 1987; Frischer et al., 1992). Although the review was rather short for such a complex issue, it did refer to a number of important possibilities of confounding that need to be controlled for, including socio-economic status, active smoking and symptom prevalence in parents.

For each of a number of studies on ETS and asthma published by 1992, the US EPA report *"Respiratory health effects of passive smoking: lung cancer and other disorders"* (National Cancer Institute, 1993) presented a paragraph summarizing the results. These included only four studies relevant to asthma exacerbation (Evans et al., 1987; O'Connor et al., 1987; Murray and Morrison, 1989; Ehrlich et al., 1992). The EPA report concluded: *"There is now sufficient evidence to conclude that passive smoking is causally associated with additional episodes and increased severity of asthma in children who already have the disease. Several studies have found that bronchial responsiveness is more prevalent and more intense among asthmatic children exposed to maternal smoke. Emergency room visits are more frequent in children of smoking mothers, and these children also have been found to need more medication for their asthma than do children of nonsmoking mothers."* Since one of the studies cited showed no significant relationships with ETS exposure (Ehrlich et al., 1992), one was extremely small (O'Connor et al., 1987), and one reported a significant relationship with only one of a range of endpoints studied (Evans et al., 1987), these conclusions seem unjustified based on this limited evidence.

A short review of *"passive smoking in childhood"* (Di Benedetto, 1995) included a section on *"asthma and bronchial responsiveness."* The author stated that *"it is well known that maternal cigarette smoking aggravates asthma symptoms and bronchial responsiveness in children with an established diagnosis of the disease,"* citing associations with increased use of health services, asthma medications and asthma symptoms. No references were cited and the review was very far from comprehensive. The author noted that *"the mechanisms by which passive smoking might increase bronchial responsiveness is still unclear"* and it is possible that *"children exposed to passive smoking might exhibit an increased risk of acquiring severe viral infections, which might cause bronchial hyperresponsiveness."*

The California EPA report *"Health effects of exposure to environmental tobacco smoke"* (National Cancer Institute, 1999) reviewed epidemiologic evidence on asthma exacerbation in children, reaching the conclusion that

> "The studies reviewed ... support the previous finding by the U.S. EPA (1992) that there is 'sufficient evidence ... that passive smoking is causally associated with additional episodes and increased severity of asthma in children who already have the disease.'"

The main body of the section consisted of mini-reviews of studies identified by them as relevant. They failed to mention some early studies we cite (including O'Connell and Logan, 1974; Gortmaker et al., 1982; Aderele, 1982; Fergusson and Horwood, 1985; Martinez et al., 1988; Weitzman et al., 1990a; Weitzman et al., 1990b; Frischer et al., 1992; Frischer et al., 1993) as well as any study published between 1995 and 1997, with one exception (Strachan and Carey, 1995), so missing eight studies we consider (Chan and Chen, 1995; LeSon and Gershwin, 1995; Jindal et al., 1996; MacArthur et al., 1996; Meijer et al., 1996; Abulhosn et al., 1997; Hu et al., 1997; Callén Blecua et al., 1997). While the report generally summarized the results of the studies accurately enough, they were uncritical as they failed to detect obvious flaws we have noted in section 5.1. These include the failure to properly investigate interactions with age and sex in the third Vancouver paper (Murray and Morrison, 1989) and to detect the lack of association with ETS exposure in the second half of the Vancouver study (Murray and Morrison, 1993).

The review also had some strange statements. These included the unsound view that the Denver study (Ostro et al., 1994) which *"had more than 10,000 observations, ... afforded substantial power to detect associations with indoor exposures, including ETS."* But power depends mainly on the number of subjects, and only 164 asthmatics were studied! Also, having described the Sheffield study (Strachan and Carey, 1995) they concluded that *"This study examines risk factors for having severe asthma versus not having asthma at all; it does not address whether exposure to ETS or other factors influence the severity of asthma among children who already have the disease."* If so, why include it in the section? In fact, one can extract relevant data (see section 5.1.4), but these are not the data they cited. Where associations were not seen, comments were often made about lack of power and of possible underestimation of effects due to misclassification of exposure. The section contained no discussion whatsoever of any potential sources of possible bias. Nor did it contain any linking paragraphs between the mini-reviews and the conclusion to describe how the conclusion was reached. As such, the section was totally one-sided and unscientific, and provided no valid support for its conclusions.

Of a series of papers on effects of parental smoking on the respiratory health of children published in Thorax by the group from St George's Hospital Medical School, two dealt specifically with data on asthma exacerbation.

The first, entitled *"Parental smoking and childhood asthma: longitudinal and case-control studies"* (Strachan and Cook, 1998a), reviewed epidemiological studies in healthy children as well as in asthmatics. It concluded that:

> "The excess incidence of wheezing in smoking households appears to be largely non-atopic 'wheezy bronchitis' with a relatively benign prognosis, but among children with established asthma, parental smoking is associated with more severe disease. This apparent paradox may be reconciled if environmental tobacco smoke is considered a co-factor provoking wheezing attacks, rather than a cause of the underlying asthmatic tendency."

Elsewhere in the paper it makes it clear that the mechanism postulated is that ETS is a co-factor *"operating with intercurrent infections."*

They summarized data from 13 studies of asthma severity and stated that *"due to the different approaches employed in each study, no formal meta-analysis is possible"* (a view one cannot dissent from), but a *"qualitative review ... suggests greater disease severity in children exposed to smoking in the household, a pattern which is more consistent among asthmatics attending hospital as outpatients or inpatients than among cases identified through population surveys."* They also commented on the lack of adjustment for potential confounding in these studies and considered that *"some of the associations of parental smoking with health service utilisation, in particular, may reflect a common association with lower socio-economic status."* They also noted that the striking association of intubation with ETS exposure seen in the Davis study (LeSon and Gershwin, 1995) *"was stronger than that with a range of psychosocial variables, suggesting that it would not be entirely explained by socio-economic confounding."*

This review (Strachan and Cook, 1998b) also noted that the results of the early Minnesota study (O'Connell and Logan, 1974) are difficult to interpret. It also highlighted the change in the relationship between maternal smoking and asthma severity before and after July 1986 seen in the Vancouver study (Murray and Morrison, 1993). Like us, they are unconvinced by the authors' claim that this is due to an alteration in parental smoking habits following advice from clinicians to avoid smoking in the home or in the presence of the child, noting that this claim is based only on anecdotal reports and not on objective evidence.

The second relevant paper from the St George's Hospital Medical School Group, entitled *"Parental smoking, bronchial reactivity and peak flow variability in children"* (Cook and Strachan, 1998), concluded that *"A clear effect of exposure to environmental tobacco smoke on BHR in the general population has not been established. While the meta-analysis suggests a small but real increase in BHR in school aged children, it seems likely that this estimate is biased upwards due to publication bias. In contrast, limited evidence suggests greater variation in peak expiratory flow in children of smoking parents."*

These conclusions were mainly based on data for healthy children. Though some studies of asthmatics were cited, these were not clearly separated out in the tables summarizing the results. The authors noted that of five studies of the effect of ETS on bronchial hyperresponsiveness in asthmatic or wheezing subjects compared with normal subjects, two reported a stronger effect in asthmatics (O'Connor et al., 1987; Martinez et al., 1988), two reported a stronger effect in non-asthmatics (Strachan et al., 1990; Frischer et al., 1992) and one reported a similar association (Agudo et al., 1994). We have included only three of these five studies (O'Connor et al., 1987; Martinez et al., 1988; Frischer et al., 1992) in our review, the other two (Strachan et al., 1990; Agudo et al., 1994) being rejected for reasons discussed in section 5.1. The authors also noted a lack of significant association in asthmatic children with ETS exposure for peak variability (Frischer et al., 1993).

While the St George's Hospital Medical School reviews were relatively thorough, they gave little attention to the problem of confounding. Since their proposed mechanism hinged around ETS acting as a co-factor operating with intercurrent infection, it is all the more surprising that the authors have apparently not investigated at all the possibility of bias if exposure to infections is greater in households with smokers, given the increased proneness of smokers to infections of various types (Arcavi and Benowitz, 2004). There was also no emphasis on the absence of data to distinguish potential effects of maternal smoking in pregnancy and of ETS exposure.

Another review was entitled *"Environmental tobacco smoke, indoor allergens, and childhood asthma"* (Gold, 2000). A brief section on *"ETS and exacerbation of asthma"* referred to previous reviews (National Cancer Institute, 1993; Strachan and Cook, 1998a) and to only a few of the relevant studies (Evans et al., 1987; O'Connor et al., 1987; Murray and Morrison, 1989). It highlighted the importance of acute respiratory infections in the exacerbation of asthma, but did not mention the problem of lack of control for such infections in the ETS studies. Nor were the difficulties of distinguishing ETS and *in utero* exposure discussed.

The review concluded that ETS *"can exacerbate already established childhood asthma."*

A review on *"Environmental tobacco smoke and respiratory diseases"* (Jaakkola, 2000) included in its section on *"Severity of asthma"* a paragraph mainly summarizing the findings of other major reviews (Strachan and Cook, 1998a; National Cancer Institute, 1999). The author noted that *"due to highly variable outcomes, a formal meta-analysis was not possible to carry out,"* and concluded that *"several studies carried out all over the world provide strong evidence that ETS exposure is related to a more severe form of asthma and poor overall control of asthma in children ≤17 years."* The review summarized much of the available data on bronchial hyperresponsiveness and PEF variability, though when considering *"ventilatory lung function"* effects in asthmatics were not separated out. In the summary the author stated that *"Parental smoking causes asthma in children, and the evidence strongly supports its role in aggravating asthmatic symptoms."*

As noted in Chapter 4, the updated report of the California EPA (California EPA, 2005) included asthma exacerbation in adults in their list of *"Effects Causally Associated with ETS Exposure."* The same conclusion was reached for children. They described studies in children published since their original report (National Cancer Institute, 1999). Of these we rejected two (Willers et al., 2000; Gilliland et al., 2003) as the endpoint was not asthma, but the rest are considered in this report (MacArthur et al., 1996; Meijer et al., 1996; Abulhosn et al., 1997; Dubus et al., 1998; Oddoze et al., 1999; Schwartz et al., 2000; Li et al., 2000; Crombie et al., 2001; Ehrlich et al., 2001; Venners et al., 2001; Melén et al., 2001; Mannino et al., 2002). As with the original California EPA report (National Cancer Institute, 1999), many relevant references were missed. Even restricting attention to those epidemiological studies of asthma exacerbation and severity published between 1998 and 2002 which one would have expected to appear in the update, there were 15 omissions (Seidler et al., 1998; Wafula et al., 1999; Shamssain and Shamsian, 1999; El-Dahr et al., 2000; Güler et al., 2000; Ratageri et al., 2000; Gürkan et al., 2000; Al-Ghamdy et al., 2000; Mayo, 2001; Wilson et al., 2001a; Morkjaroenpong et al., 2002; Gaspar et al., 2002; Kalaajieh, 2002; Wamboldt et al., 2002; Dales et al., 2002), as against only the seven they considered. Clearly, their literature searching was inadequate.

While short summaries of the 14 new studies were included, the discussion and interpretation was very limited, the relevant section being reproduced below:

> "Taken together, the recent evidence supports the original 1997 Cal/EPA report's conclusion that ETS is a causal factor for asthma exacerbation among

children. The cross-sectional studies are all limited by the possibility of selection effects, such as smoking reduction by parents who have children with more severe asthma. This bias, which is unavoidable in cross-sectional studies, would attenuate any observed risk estimate. The longitudinal studies, which are less prone to this bias, are most consistent with an adverse effect of ETS on childhood asthma status, and consistently show elevated risk of symptoms, more and prolonged medication use, and increased school absenteeism. In addition, as shown in a recent meta-analysis by Vork *et al.*, (2002), hidden environmental differences between studies may distort risk estimates. Specifically, higher ETS-related asthma risks were reported in areas with lower ambient air pollution. It was suggested that in polluted areas, individuals who are genetically more susceptible to asthma may be more affected by the ambient air pollution than by ETS, thus masking the effects of ETS exposure. If nondifferential, failure to account for the effects of ambient air pollution could bias risk estimates towards unity."

The report lacked any attempt to bring together all the relevant data relating to specific endpoints, so provided no good information on the consistency of the findings.

3.3. Conclusions

There are quite a substantial number of studies in asthmatic children which, taken together, suggest strongly that ETS exposure increases the risk of acute exacerbations. However the results are heterogeneous, and interpretation of the association is not completely straightforward, with failure to control for potential confounding variables, including maternal smoking in pregnancy. An effect on reduced lung function may exist, with the results most suggestive for $FEF_{25\text{-}75\%}$, but has not been clearly established. There is no consistent association of bronchial responsiveness with ETS exposure.

REFERENCES

Abulhosn, R. S., Morray, B. H., Lewellyn, C. E., and Redding, G. J. (1995). Effects of passive smoking on recovery following hospitalization of children with acute asthma (Abstract). *Pediatr. Res.* 37, 387A.

Abulhosn, R. S., Morray, B. H., Llewellyn, C. E., and Redding, G. J. (1997). Passive smoke exposure impairs recovery after hospitalization for acute asthma. *Arch. Pediatr. Adolesc. Med.* 151, 135-139.

Aderele, W. I. (1982). Aetiologic, precipitating and environmental factors in childhood asthma. *Niger. J. Paediatr.* 9, 26-31.

Agudo, A., Bardagi, S., Romero, P. V., and González, C. A. (1994). Exercise-induced airways narrowing and exposure to environmental tobacco smoke in schoolchildren. *Am. J. Epidemiol.* 140, 409-417.

Al-Ghamdy, Y. S., Al-Haddad, N. S., Adelgadir, M. H., Qureshi, N. A., Saleh, M. A., and Khalil, M. M. (2000). Socioclinical profile of children with asthma in Al-Majmaah Health Province. *Saudi Med. J.* 21, 847-851.

Arcavi, L., and Benowitz, N. L. (2004). Cigarette smoking and infection. *Arch. Intern. Med.* 164, 2206-2216.

Bayona, M., Montealegre, F., Gomes de Andrade, V. L., and Treviño, F. (2002). Prognostic factors of severe asthma in Puerto Rico. *P. R. Health Sci. J.* 21, 213-219.

Bener, A., Al-Frayh, A. R., and Al-Jawadi, T. Q. (1991). Parental smoking and the risk of childhood asthma. *J. Asthma* 28, 281-286.

California Environmental Protection Agency. (2005). *Proposed identification of environmental tobacco smoke as a toxic air contaminant - as approved by the Scientific Review Panel on June 24, 2005.* Available from: *www.arb.ca.gov/toxics/ets/finalreport/finalreport.htm*

Callén Blecua, M., González Pérez-Yarza, E., Garmendia Iglesias, A., Mintegui Aranburu, J., and Emparanza Knörr, J. I. (1997). Efecto del tabaquismo pasivo sobre la función pulmonar del niño asmatico (Effect of passive smoking on pulmonary function in the asthmatic child). *An. Esp. Pediatr.* 47, 383-388.

Canadian Paediatric Society (1986). Secondhand cigarette smoke worsens symptoms in children with asthma. *CMAJ* 135, 321-323.

Chadwick, S. (1996). The impact of asthma in an inner city general practice. *Child Care Health Dev.* 22, 175-186.

Chan, C. C., and Chen, S. J. (1995). The influence of environmental tobacco smoke (ETS) exposure on asthmatic children's peak expiratory flow (PEF) (Abstract). Presented at the Annual Conference of the International Society for Environmental Epidemiology and the International Society for Exposure Analysis, Noordwijkerhout, The Netherlands, August 30 - September 1, 1995. *Epidemiology* 6, 13S.

Chapman, R. S., Hadden, W. C., and Perlin, S. A. (2003). Influences of asthma and household environment on lung function in children and adolescents. The Third National Health and Nutrition Examination Survey. *Am. J. Epidemiol.* 158, 175-189.

Chilmonczyk, B. A., Salmun, L. M., Megathlin, K. N., Neveux, L. M., Palomaki, G. E., Knight, G. J., Pulkkinen, A. J., and Haddow, J. E. (1993). Association between exposure to environmental tobacco smoke and exacerbations of asthma in children. *N. Engl. J. Med.* 328, 1665-1669.

Cook, D. G., and Strachan, D. P. (1998). Parental smoking, bronchial reactivity and peak flow variability in children. *Thorax* 53, 295-301.

Crombie, I. K., Wright, A. I. L., Clark, R. A., and Slane, P. W. (2001). Does passive smoking increase the frequency of health service contacts in children with asthma? *Thorax* 56, 9-12.

Dahms, T. E., Bolin, J. F., and Slavin, R. G. (1981). Passive smoking: Effects on bronchial asthma. *Chest* 80, 530-534.

Dales, R. E., Choi, B., Chen, Y., and Tang, M. (2002). Influence of family income on hospital visits for asthma among Canadian school children. *Thorax* 57, 513-517.

Di Benedetto, G. (1995). Passive smoking in childhood. *J. R. Soc. Health* 115, 13-16.

Dubus, J.-C., Oddoze, C., Badier, M., Guillot, C., and Bruguerolle, B. (1998). Possible interaction between exposure to environmental tobacco smoke and therapy in children with asthma. *Clin. Sci.* 95, 143-149.

Ehrlich, R., Jordaan, E., du Toit, D., Potter, P., Volmink, J., Zwarenstein, M., and Weinberg, E. (2001). Household smoking and bronchial hyperresponsiveness in children with asthma. *J. Asthma* 38, 239-251.

Ehrlich, R., Kattan, M., Godbold, J., Saltzberg, D. S., Grimm, K. T., Landrigan, P. J., and Lilienfeld, D. E. (1992). Childhood asthma and passive smoking: Urinary cotinine as a biomarker of exposure. *Am. Rev. Respir. Dis.* 145, 594-599.

Ehrlich, R., Kattan, M., and Lilienfeld, D. E. (1993). Is passive smoking a cause of asthma in childhood? *J. Smoking-Related Dis.* 4, 91-99.

El-Dahr, J., Armstrong, M., McCants, M., Gibson, R., Rando, R., Myers, L., Romalewski, C., and Lehrer, S. (2000). Improved lung function and symptoms in response to decreased exposure to parental smoking in children with asthma (Abstract). Presented at American Academy of Allergy Asthma and Immunology (AAAAI) 56th Annual Meeting, San Diego, California, USA. March 3-8, 2000. *J. Allergy Clin. Immunol.* 105(1 part 2), S81, abstract number 245.

Evans, D., Levison, M. J., Feldman, C. H., Clark, N. M., Wasilewski, Y., Levin, B., and Mellins, R. B. (1987). The impact of passive smoking on emergency room visits of urban children with asthma. *Am. Rev. Respir. Dis.* 135, 567-572.

Fergusson, D. M., and Horwood, L. J. (1985). Parental smoking and respiratory illness during early childhood: a six-year longitudinal study. *Pediatr. Pulmonol.* 1, 99-106.

Fielder, H. M. P., Lyons, R. A., Heaven, M., Morgan, H., Govier, P., and Hooper, M. (1999). Effect of environmental tobacco smoke on peak flow variability. *Arch. Dis. Child.* 80, 253-256.

Frischer, T., Kuehr, J., Meinert, R., Karmaus, W., Barth, R., Hermann-Kunz, E., and Urbanek, R. (1992). Maternal smoking in early childhood: a risk factor for bronchial responsiveness to exercise in primary-school children. *J. Pediatr.* 121, 17-22.

Frischer, T., Kühr, J., Meinert, R., Karmaus, W., and Urbanek, R. (1993). Influence of maternal smoking on variability of peak expiratory flow rate in school children. *Chest* 104, 1133-1137.

Gaspar, A. P., Morais-Almeida, M. A., Pires, G. C., Prates, S. R., Câmara, R. A., Godinho, N. M., Arêde, C. S., and Rosado-Pinto, J. E. (2002). Risk factors for asthma admissions in children. *Allergy Asthma Proc.* 23, 295-301.

Gilliland, F. D., Berhane, K., Islam, T., Wenten, M., Rappaport, E., Avol, E., Gauderman, W. J., McConnell, R., and Peters, J. M. (2003). Environmental tobacco smoke and absenteeism related to respiratory illness in schoolchildren. *Am. J. Epidemiol.* 157, 861-869.

Gilliland, F. D., Li, Y.-F., and Peters, J. M. (2001). Effects of maternal smoking during pregnancy and environmental tobacco smoke on asthma and wheezing in children. *Am. J. Respir. Crit. Care Med.* 163, 429-436.

Gold, D. R. (2000). Environmental tobacco smoke, indoor allergens, and childhood asthma. *Environ. Health Perspect.* 108, 643-651.

Gortmaker, S. L., Walker, D. K., Jacobs, F. H., and Ruch-Ross, H. (1982). Parental smoking and the risk of childhood asthma. *Am. J. Public Health* 72, 574-579.

Güler, G., Önes, Ü., Kiliç, A., and Tamay, Z. (2000). The effect of exposure to environmental tobacco smoke on clinical findings in asthmatic schoolchildren (Abstract). Presented at American Academy of Allergy Asthma and Immunology (AAAAI) 56th Annual Meeting, San Diego, California, USA. March 3-8, 2000. *J. Allergy Clin. Immunol.* 105(1 Pt 2), S125, abstract number 375.

Gürkan, F., Ace, A., Haspolat, K., Derman, O., and Bosmak, M. (2000). Predictors for multiple hospital admissions in children with asthma. *Can. Respir. J.* 7, 163-166.

Halterman, J. S., Szilagyi, P. G., Yoos, H. L., Conn, K. M., Kaczorowski, J. M., Holzhauer, R. J., Lauver, S. C., Neely, T. L., Callahan, P. M., and McConnochie, K. M. (2004). Benefits of a school-based asthma treatment program in the absence of secondhand smoke exposure: results of a randomized clinical trial. *Arch. Pediatr. Adolesc. Med.* 158, 460-467.

Henderson, F. W., Henry, M. M., Ivins, S. S., Morris, R., Neebe, E. C., Leu, S.-Y., Stewart, P. W., and The Physicians of Raleigh Pediatric Associates PA. (1995). Correlates of recurrent wheezing in school-age children. *Am. J. Respir. Crit. Care Med.* 151, 1786-1793.

Hu, F. B., Persky, V., Flay, B. R., Zelli, A., Cooksey, J., and Richardson, J. (1997). Prevalence of asthma and wheezing in public schoolchildren: association with maternal smoking during pregnancy. *Ann. Allergy Asthma Immunol.* 79, 80-84.

Huss, K., Rand, C. S., Butz, A. M., Eggleston, P. A., Murigande, C., Thompson, L. C., Schneider, S., Weeks, K., and Malveaux, F. J. (1994). Home environmental risk factors in urban minority asthmatic children. *Ann. Allergy* 72, 173-177.

Jaakkola, M. S. (2000). Environmental tobacco smoke and respiratory diseases. In I. Annesi-maesano, A. Gulsvik, and G. Viegi (Eds.), *Respiratory epidemiology in Europe* (pp. 322-383). (European Respiratory Society Monograph no 15.) Sheffield, UK: European Respiratory Society.

Jindal, S. K., Gupta, D., Chattopadhya, S., and Kumar, L. (1996). Recent exposure to environmental tobacco smoke (ETS) precipitates acute attack in non-smoker asthmatics (Abstract). Presented at Chest 1996 World Congress, San Francisco, California, October 27-31, 1996. *Chest* 110(4 Suppl), 89S.

Kalaajieh, W. K. (2002). Factors associated with recurrent hospitalizations in asthmatic children. *Rev. Fr. Allergol. Immunol. Clin.* 42, 640-644.

Karadag, B., Karakoç, F., Ceran, O., Ersu, R., Inan, S., and Dagli, E. (2003). Does passive smoke exposure trigger acute asthma attack in children? *Allergol. Immunopathol.* 31, 318-323.

Lebowitz, M. D. (1984a). Influence of passive smoking on pulmonary function: a survey. *Prev. Med.* 13, 645-655.

Lebowitz, M. D. (1984b). The effects of environmental tobacco smoke exposure and gas stoves on daily peak flow rates in asthmatic and non-asthmatic families. *Eur. J. Respir. Dis.* 65(Suppl 133), 90-97.

Lee, P. N. (1988). Misclassification of smoking habits and passive smoking. A review of the evidence. *Int. Arch. Occup. Environ. Health* (Suppl), 1-103. Heidelberg: Springer-Verlag.

Lee, P.N., and Forey, B.A. (2007). The role of environmental tobacco smoke in asthma induction and exacerbation in children and adults. Nova Science Publishers, Inc. New York.

LeSon, S., and Gershwin, M. E. (1995). Risk factors for asthmatic patients requiring intubation. I. Observations in children. *J. Asthma* 32, 285-294.

Li, Y.-F., Gilliland, F. D., Berhane, K., McConnell, R., Gauderman, W. J., Rappaport, E. B., and Peters, J. M. (2000). Effects of *in utero* and environmental tobacco smoke exposure on lung function in boys and girls with and without asthma. *Am. J. Respir. Crit. Care Med.* 162, 2097-2104.

Lilienfeld, D. E., Ehrlich, R. I., Kattan, M., Saltzber, D. S., Grimm, K. T., and Landrigan, P. J. (1990). Passive smoking and urinary cotinine levels in acute and non-acute asthmatics. (Abstract) In *Abstracts of International Epidemiological Association Twelth Scientific Meeting* (p. 78, abstract number 332). (90024-1772.) Los Angeles, CA: International Epidemiological Association.

MacArthur, C., Calpin, C., Parkin, P. C., and Feldman, W. (1996). Factors associated with pediatric asthma readmissions. *J. Allergy Clin. Immunol.* 98, 992-993.

Mannino, D. M., Homa, D. M., and Redd, S. C. (2002). Involuntary smoking and asthma severity in children: data from the Third National Health and Nutrition Examination Survey. *Chest* 122, 409-415.

Martinez, F. D., Antognoni, G., Macri, F., Bonci, E., Midulla, F., de Castro, G., and Ronchetti, R. (1988). Parental smoking enhances bronchial responsiveness in nine-year-old children. *Am. Rev. Respir. Dis.* 138, 518-523.

Mayo, P. R. (2001). Effect of passive smoking on theophylline clearance in children. *Ther. Drug Monit.* 23, 503-505.

Meijer, G. G., Postma, D. S., van der Heide, S., De Reus, D. M., Roorda, R. J., Koëter, G. H., and Van Aalderen, M. C. (1996). Exogenous stimuli and circadian peak expiratory flow variation in allergic asthmatic children. *Am. J. Respir. Crit. Care Med.* 153, 237-242.

Meinert, R., Frischer, T., and Kuehr, J. (1994). The "healthy passive smoker": relationship between bronchial hyper-reactivity in school children and maternal smoking. *J. Epidemiol. Community Health* 48, 325-326.

Melén, E., Nordvall, L., van Hage-Hamsten, M., Wickman, M., and Lindfors, A. (2000). Causes of severe asthma in preschool children (Abstract). Presented at American Academy of Allergy Asthma and Immunology (AAAAI) 56th Annual Meeting, San Diego, California, USA. March 3-8, 2000. *J. Allergy Clin. Immunol.* 105 (1 Pt 2), S80, abstract number 242.

Melén, E., Wickman, M., Nordvall, S. L., van Hage-Hamsten, M., and Lindfors, A. (2001). Influence of early and current environmental exposure factors on sensitization and outcome of asthma in pre-school children. *Allergy* 56, 646-652.

Morgan, W. J., Crain, E. F., Gruchalla, R. S., O'Connor, G. T., Kattan, M., Evans, R., III, Stout, J., Malindzak, G., Smartt, E., Plaut, M., Walter, M., Vaughn, B., and Mitchell, H. (2004). Results of a home-based environmental intervention among urban children with asthma. *N. Engl. J. Med.* 351, 1068-1080.

Morkjaroenpong, V., Rand, C. S., Butz, A. M., Huss, K., Eggleston, P., Malveaux, F. J., and Bartlett, S. J. (2002). Environmental tobacco smoke exposure and nocturnal symptoms among inner-city children with asthma. *J. Allergy Clin. Immunol.* 110, 147-153.

Murray, A. B., and Morrison, B. J. (1986). The effect of cigarette smoke from the mother on bronchial responsiveness and severity of symptoms in children with asthma. *J. Allergy Clin. Immunol.* 77, 575-581.

Murray, A. B., and Morrison, B. J. (1988). Passive smoking and the seasonal difference of severity of asthma in children. *Chest* 94, 701-708.

Murray, A. B., and Morrison, B. J. (1989). Passive smoking by asthmatics: its greater effect on boys than on girls and on older than on younger children. *Pediatrics* 84, 451-459.

Murray, A. B., and Morrison, B. J. (1992). Effect of passive smoking on asthmatic children who have and who have not had atopic dermatitis. *Chest* 101, 16-18.

Murray, A. B., and Morrison, B. J. (1993). The decrease in severity of asthma in children of parents who smoke since the parents have been exposing them to less cigarette smoke. *J. Allergy Clin. Immunol.* 91, 102-110.

National Cancer Institute. Shopland, D. R. (Ed.) (1993). *Respiratory health effects of passive smoking: lung cancer and other disorders. The report of the US Environmental Protection Agency. Smoking and Tobacco Control. Monograph No. 4.* (NIH Pub. No. 93-3605.) Bethesda, MD: US Department of Health and Human Services, Public Health Service, National Institutes of Health.

National Cancer Institute. Shopland, D. R., Zeise, L., and Dunn, A. (Eds.) (1999). *Health effects of exposure to environmental tobacco smoke. The report of the California Environmental Protection Agency. Smoking and Tobacco Control. Monograph No. 10.* (NIH Pub. No. 99-4645.) Bethesda, MD: US Department of Health and Human Services, National Institutes of Health, National Cancer Institute. Available from: *http://cancercontrol.cancer.gov/tcrb/monographs/10/index.html*

O'Connell, E. J., and Logan, G. B. (1974). Parental smoking in childhood asthma. *Ann. Allergy* 32, 142-145.

O'Connor, G. T., Weiss, S. T., Tager, I. B., and Speizer, F. E. (1987). The effect of passive smoking on pulmonary function and nonspecific bronchial responsiveness in a population-based sample of children and young adults. *Am. Rev. Respir. Dis.* 135, 800-804. Erratum appears in *Am. Rev. Resp. Dis.* 1987,136, 532.

Oddoze, C., Dubus, J. C., Badier, M., Thirion, X., Pauli, A. M., Pastor, J., and Bruguerolle, B. (1999). Urinary cotinine and exposure to parental smoking in a population of children with asthma. *Clin. Chem.* 45, 505-509.

Ogborn, C. J., Duggan, A. K., and DeAngelis, C. (1994). Urinary cotinine as a measure of passive smoke exposure in asthmatic children. *Clin. Pediatr.* 33, 220-226.

Ostro, B. D., Lipsett, M. J., Mann, J. K., Wiener, M. B., and Selner, J. (1994). Indoor air pollution and asthma: results from a panel study. *Am. J. Respir. Crit. Care Med.* 149, 1400-1406.

Ratageri, V. H., Kabra, S. K., Dwivedi, S. N., and Seth, V. (2000). Factors associated with severe asthma. *Indian Pediatr.* 37, 1072-1082.

Salmun, L. M., Chilmonczyk, B. A., Megathlin, K. N., Neveux, L. M., Knight, G. J., Pulkkinen, A. J., and Haddow, J. E. (1992). The extent and impact of environmental tobacco smoke (ETS) exposure in children with asthma (Abstract). *J. Allergy Clin. Immunol.* 89, 231.

Schwartz, J., Timonen, K. L., and Pekkanen, J. (2000). Respiratory effects of environmental tobacco smoke in a panel study of asthmatic and symptomatic children. *Am. J. Respir. Crit. Care Med.* 161, 802-806.

Seidler, A., Schlaud, M., Raum, E., and Schwartz, F. W. (1998). Prädiktoren der Verlaufsentwicklung asthmatischer Beschwerden im frühen Kindesalter - Ergebnisse einer Follow-up-Untersuchung. (Predictors of the course of obstructive airways disorders in children - results of a follow-up study). *Klin. Padiatr.* 210, 24-29.

Shamssain, M. H., and Shamsian, N. (1999). Prevalence and severity of asthma, rhinitis, and atopic eczema: the north east study. *Arch. Dis. Child.* 81, 313-317.

Soussan, D., Liard, R., Zureik, M., Touron, D., Rogeaux, Y., and Neukirch, F. (2003). Treatment compliance, passive smoking, and asthma control: a three year cohort study. *Arch. Dis. Child.* 88, 229-233.

Speer, F. (1968). Tobacco and the nonsmoker. A study of subjective symptoms. *Arch. Environ. Health* 16, 443-446.

Strachan, D. P., and Carey, I. M. (1995). Home environment and severe asthma in adolescence: a population based case-control study. *BMJ* 311, 1053-1056.

Strachan, D. P., and Cook, D. G. (1998a). Parental smoking and childhood asthma: longitudinal and case-control studies. *Thorax* 53, 204-212.

Strachan, D. P., and Cook, D. G. (1998b). Parental smoking, middle ear disease and adenotonsillectomy in children. *Thorax* 53, 50-56.

Strachan, D. P., Jarvis, M. J., and Feyerabend, C. (1990). The relationship of salivary cotinine to respiratory symptoms, spirometry, and exercise-induced bronchospasm in seven-year-old children. *Am. Rev. Respir. Dis.* 142, 147-151.

Tarlo, S. M., Broder, I., Corey, P., Chan-Yeung, M., Ferguson, A., Becker, A., Warren, P., Simons, F. E. R., Sherlock, C., Okada, M., and Manfreda, J. (2000). A case-control study of the role of cold symptoms and other historical triggering factors in asthma exacerbations. *Can. Respir. J.* 7, 42-48.

Toyoshima, K., Hayashida, M., Yasunami, J., Takamatsu, I., Niwa, H., and Muraoka, T. (1987). Factors influencing the prognosis of wheezy infants. *J. Asthma* 24, 267-270.

Venners, S. A., Wang, X., Chen, C., Wang, B., Ni, J., Jin, Y., Yang, J., Fang, Z., Weiss, S. T., and Xu, X. (2001). Exposure-response relationship between paternal smoking and children's pulmonary function. *Am. J. Respir. Crit. Care Med.* 164, 973-976.

Vork, K. L., Broadwin, R. L., and Lipsett, M. J. (2002). Household environmental tobacco smoke (ETS) exposure and risk of childhood asthma - techniques to reduce between-study heterogeneity in a meta-analysis. In *Indoor Air 2002*, Vol. 2, Proceedings of 9th International Conference on Indoor Air Quality and Climate, Monterey California, June 30 -July 5 2002 (pp. 483-488).

Wafula, E. M., Limbe, M. S., Onyango, F. E., and Nduati, R. (1999). Effects of passive smoking and breastfeeding on childhood bronchial asthma. *East Afr. Med. J.* 76, 606-609.

Wamboldt, F. S., Jo, J., Milgrom, H., Wamboldt, M. Z., Sanders, B., Szefler, S. J., and Bender, B. G. (2002). Prevalence and correlates of household exposures to tobacco smoke and pets in children with asthma. *J. Pediatr.* 141, 109-115.

Weitzman, M., Gortmaker, S., and Sobol, A. (1990a). Racial, social, and environmental risks for childhood asthma. *Am. J. Dis. Child.* 144, 1189-1194.

Weitzman, M., Gortmaker, S., Walker, D. K., and Sobol, A. (1990b). Maternal smoking and childhood asthma. *Pediatrics* 85, 505-511.

Willers, S., Axmon, A., Feyerabend, C., Nielsen, J., Skarping, G., and Skerfving, S. (2000). Assessment of environmental tobacco smoke exposure in children with asthmatic symptoms by questionnaire and cotinine concentrations in plasma, saliva, and urine. *J. Clin. Epidemiol.* 53, 715-721.

Wilson, K., Clark, H., Hotz, S., and Dent, R. (2001a). Impact of smoking status on weight loss and cardiovascular risk factors. *J. Epidemiol. Community Health* 55, 213-214.

Wilson, S. R., Yamada, E. G., Sudhakar, R., Roberto, L., Mannino, D., Mejia, C., and Huss, N. (2001b). A controlled trial of an environmental tobacco smoke reduction intervention in low-income children with asthma. *Chest* 120, 1709-1722.

Wood, P. R., Hidalgo, H. A., Prihoda, T. J., and Kromer, M. E. (1993). Hispanic children with asthma: morbidity. *Pediatrics* 91, 62-69.

ACKNOWLEDGEMENTS

We thank John Fry for helpful comments, Katharine Coombs for data entry, Pauline Wassell and Diana Morris for their patient and accurate word processing, and Yvonne Cooper for obtaining and maintaining the literature. We are grateful to Philip Morris International, which gave financial support to the publication of this review, and to other tobacco companies which supported preliminary work on asthma. The preparation of all stages of the book, including interpretation of the findings, were carried out independently of the sponsors.

INDEX

A

B

C

D

E

F

M

N

O

P

Q

R

- S -

- T -

- U -

- V -

- W -

- Y -